PHYSICIAN CAREER GUIDEBOOK

VOLUME 1

The Road to Residency
and Beyond

*What they didn't teach
you in medical school*

Sheri L. Clarke, PhD
with
Jodie Chant, MPA
&
Rebecca Kraus, PCC

ISBN-13: 9781708684631

Cover by: Cassandra Clarke
Cover photo: Masintos @Pixabay [CC0 1.0 Universal Public Domain Dedication]

This is the first book in a series titled *Physician Career Guidebook*. Books in this series are:

- *The Road to Residency and Beyond – What They Didn't Teach You in Medical School.*
- *Navigating the Chasm from Residency to Practicing Physician* (Summer 2020)
- *The Physician Influencer - Inspiring Others in the World of Medicine* (Autumn 2020)

In the future, watch for a series titled *Physician Career Reference* where we will go into more detail on subjects discussed in the *Physician Career Guidebooks*.

Acknowledgements

This book is dedicated to all of you who entered medical school with altruistic goals to improve the health and wellbeing of your patients. You have devoted yourselves to years of studying, little sleep, hard work, and plenty of student loan payments. You still have a long journey ahead of you and we would like to give you the information to be successful in your pursuits. The information you learn here will not be in your medical school curriculum but will provide you with advantages that have never been available to medical students before. We have your best interest in mind. This book is dedicated and written for YOU. Thank you for what you do and will do in your career.

Table of Contents

Foreword

Congratulations on knowing your future plans. You are going to be a doctor! Just deciding this pathway, and getting to where you are now, has been a huge process. You have entered medical school to become a physician and you are learning all about basic science, anatomy, and disease science. However, in order to be successful in your medical career, you need more than medical knowledge. You need to understand the medical education system and how to avoid the potholes along your path that can hurt your career. This Physician Career Guidebook series is a practical career guidebook to lead you through residency training, your first years as an attending physician, and becoming a physician leader. All items are generic across medical specialties and are meant to help bring the topics to your attention for your further contemplation. Each chapter is a mentoring or coaching session for a specific period of your training timeline. Use the information provided to further your career and to be better prepared for each step along the way. Each book is designed to be a guide for multiple years so you can use the appropriate chapters at the appropriate times.

Always read ahead, to ensure that you are prepared for the next chapter of your career.

Chapter One:
Introduction to
Graduate Medical Education

This book will guide you through some of the most difficult steps of becoming an attending physician. The information provided is from a seasoned graduate medical education administrator with experience at multiple levels of residency administration. As all residency programs and institutions are not the same, you should understand that these tips are recommended best practices and general in nature. At times, you may need to revise these guidelines to meet the needs of your program, but in general, you will find these guidelines very helpful.

What is Graduate Medical Education?

In the United States of America (USA), when you graduate with your medical degree, you cannot practice medicine independently like some other countries. Oversight of physicians is done at the State level licensing board. Each State sets their own requirements for a medical license. Many will require one or two years of postgraduate training before you can get an independent license. However, even then, you cannot have a thriving medical practice without Board Certification. With the current healthcare payment system, insurance companies can determine minimum standards for physicians that care for their members (your patients). Board certification or Board eligibility is a minimum standard for hospitals, health systems and most third-party payers. Board eligibility means that you have completed the necessary training to sit for specialty or sub-specialty board certification examinations. Board certification means that you have met the necessary training requirements to sit for your specialty or sub-specialty board examinations and have passed those examinations.

In order to become fully licensed to practice medicine AND be board certified, you must complete the necessary training for the specialty, also known as a residency program. If you wish to subspecialize after completing residency training, you would also have to complete the necessary training for the sub-specialty, commonly referred to as a fellowship. Medical school training is commonly referred to as Undergraduate Medical Education. Postgraduate training which includes residency and fellowship programs is called Graduate Medical Education.

Graduate Medical Education (GME) occurs in teaching institutions under the supervision of the Accreditation Council for Graduate Medical Education (ACGME). ACGME sets minimum standards for training of residents and fellows. Each specialty has curriculum requirements and experiences identified for programs to include in their training programs. All programs in the same specialty must meet these minimum standards but have flexibility on how they provide this training. When you are considering programs for the purpose of applying, there will be many things to consider. A future chapter will discuss these differences.

With ACGME, all training programs are accredited separately, and the institution is accredited as a sponsoring institution. Another element of ACGME oversight is to ensure that the clinical learning environment is a positive one for trainees. Referred to as Clinical Learning Environment Review (CLER), this is an institutional wide site visit with the GME department and hospital administrators. CLER visits are planned for every 18 months and residents are a major part of the visit. Residents tour the visitors around the hospitals and clinics. They try to speak with as many residents as possible during their visit in the actual clinical learning environment, rather than in a conference room. While you are a resident, it is likely that you will be asked to speak with these site visitors. We will discuss what to expect in a later chapter.

The important thing to understand is that there is an extensive oversight process for all residency and fellowship training. There are specific competencies and milestones that each trainee must meet in order to graduate from the program. The timeline for meeting these competencies and milestones will be very individualized. You cannot compare yourself with your classmates as easily in residency as you would have in school. You will have different experiences at different times as your rotation schedules will vary from other residents. You need to know what expectations your program has for you and make sure you are working to meet those expectations.

Understanding the Application Process

Now that you understand what GME is and how it is strictly monitored, let us discuss how you can become part of the system. When you graduate from a USA medical school or a foreign medical school with an ECFMG certificate (more about that later), you are qualified to apply for a USA residency program. Residents are generally accepted into the programs through a matching process. The primary match is the National Residency Matching Program (nrmp.org) with results announced in March. The American Urological Association runs their own match separately with results announced in January (auanet.org). The US military match results are available in December. Some institutions choose not to participate in formal matches. For those institutions, you must apply directly to the institution and they will have self-determined timelines.

Your medical school is a great resource on how to apply through the appropriate Match for your circumstances. I'll refrain from duplicating the information they will share with you. Most of you will apply through the NRMP match, so we will discuss this Match in more detail. When the time is right, your school will contact you about setting up your application in the Electronic Residency Application System (ERAS). The ERAS application is a general application that all medical students complete to participate in a match. The application system opens in mid-September the year before you will enter the program. Residency programs begin on July 1 with orientation time usually a week or two prior. Fellowships begin July 1 or August 1. Orientation time for fellowship should be 1-2 days, depending on if you went to residency at the same institution.

Residency programs begin on July 1, with orientation time usually a week or two prior. Fellowships begin July 1 or August 1.

By the time you apply via ERAS, you will have to know what specialty and the specific programs to which you will apply. You will need to have specific documentation created prior to your application. Once you apply, the residency programs will receive your application. They filter applications based on program selection guidelines within their institution. Some programs will filter by test scores (USMLE or COMLEX-USA), dean's letters, letters of reference, medical school grades, or any number of characteristics to identify quality candidates. Then, those applications that make it through the first filter will be reviewed personally by a program representative or selection committee. If the program feels you meet their recruitment standards, you will receive an interview offer. In my experience, students have told me they interview at about 8-12 programs, often in a specific geographic region. You will interview, rank your choices, and wait for the computer matching process. Communication is very important during the recruitment season. We will discuss important tips on how to communicate with the programs in Chapter Five. Once you are matched to a program, you will be communicating with that program right away to prepare for your arrival. Now that you know the general process, let's break it down into specific steps that will make you successful.

Chapter Two:
Picking the Right Specialty

When you entered medical school, you may have known you wanted to be a [fill in the blank] (pediatrician, internist, trauma surgeon, etc.). While you are in school, you have opportunities to learn more about that specialty area of practice. Take advantage of these opportunities. Ask the right questions and speak to the right people to get all the information that you need about whether this is the path for you.

Consider other specialties as well. There is not a regularly updated and comprehensive list of all the specialty and subspecialty options that are available to you. However, the American Board of Medical Specialties (ABMS) and the American Osteopathic Association (AOA) websites are an excellent resource for considering various specialties and subspecialties that lead to Board certification. Appendix A is a list of all ACGME accredited options at the time this book was published. New specialties and combinations of specialties are developed routinely, so this may change, but it will give you as starting point. You can look at the current specialty options on their website (acgme.org). When considering a specialty, you should understand the lifestyle, academic rigor, research requirements, and much more. Learn everything you can about the specialty and make sure you speak to physicians in all stages of life within that specialty. Ask them if they would choose this specialty again. What do they like most about it? What do they like least? Do they see any major changes coming in the specialty, i.e. payments, board certification, scope of practice? How do they spend their time in a typical day? Do they have any recommendations for someone just starting out? Would you choose this specialty again, if you were choosing today?

Length of Training

In GME, each year that you are post medical school graduation is tracked as a Post-Graduate Year (PGY1, PGY2, PGY3, etc.). Post-Graduate Year (PGY) is an official term used by the federal government to track your years of training since medical school graduation. It is often concurrently used as a way of identifying the class in a training program. As in, the PGY2 class is in their second year of residency. However, this is not always ideal, because if someone transfers, takes a leave of absence, or repeats rotations, the PGY can become different from the others in their level of training. For this reason, many institutions track PGY as noted above and refer to the level of training within the program as Program Year (PRG1, PRG2, etc.) or Resident Year (R1, R2, etc.). For the purposes of our discussion, we will be using the term PGY for simplicity.

Your GME experience can take anywhere from three to nine years. Residency training is three to five years and optional fellowship training can add another three to six years to become a subspecialist. Table 1 shows the length of a few common specialties. In general, primary care specialties are known as pediatrics, family medicine, internal medicine, and obstetrics/gynecology (OB/GYN). These specialties, except for OB/GYN, are three-year residencies. OB/GYN and Anesthesiology are four-year residencies. Other surgical residencies are usually five years in length.

Table 1: Length of Residency Training

PGY 1	PGY 2	PGY 3	PGY 4	PGY 5
Emergency Medicine				
Family Medicine				
Internal Medicine				
Pediatrics				
Osteopathic Neuromusculoskeletal Medicine				
Anesthesiology				
Obstetrics and Gynecology				
Neurology				
Ophthalmology				
Pathology				
Psychiatry				
General Surgery				
Neurological Surgery				
Orthopaedic Surgery				
Otolaryngology/Facial Plastic Surgery				
Urological Surgery				
Diagnostic Radiology				

Table 2 provides some insight into subspecialty training. In order to subspecialize, you must first complete a residency program, take your specialty board examinations, and enter additional training via a fellowship. Then, you take the subspecialty board examinations.

Each subspecialty has a residency program pre-requisite. Gastroenterology and cardiology require internal medicine. Geriatrics will accept internal medicine or family medicine residency training. There are some subspecialties that require a residency and fellowship, before entering another fellowship. This is the case for interventional cardiology. You would do three years in internal medicine, three years in cardiology, and then one year in interventional cardiology. Seven years of postgraduate training in total. In order to determine the path to a subspecialty, review Appendix A. I also recommend that you find the standards for each training program on the ACGME website. In each document, you will find more information about the curriculum, required experiences, and expectations for graduation.

Table 2: Length of Fellowship Subspecialty Options

PGY 1	PGY 2	PGY 3	PGY 4	PGY 5	PGY 6
Internal Medicine			Allergy and Immunology		
Internal Medicine			Cardiology		
Internal Medicine			Gastroenterology		
Internal Medicine or Family Medicine			Geriatrics		
Internal Medicine			Hematology/Oncology		
Internal Medicine			Hematology		
Internal Medicine			Medical Oncology		
Internal Medicine			Pulmonary/Critical Care		
Internal Medicine			Pulmonary		
Internal Medicine			Critical Care		

Eligibility Considerations

When you are choosing between two specialties that have different lengths of training, there is one more thing to consider when making this decision. As with college sports, there is "eligibility" with residency. However, this eligibility is regarding funding to the hospital that trains you.

The federal government through the Centers for Medicare and Medicaid Services (www.cms.gov) pays for part of your residency training. Details about this can be found in Title 42, Chapter IV, part 4`3, subpart F, Section 413.78 of the Federal Register. It is a very complex system. Basically, each sponsoring institution can claim residents and fellows on their federal cost report. There is a limit on the number of positions that can be claimed at each institution. Most sponsoring institutions fill more residency positions than they can claim for reimbursement. In addition, the amount of reimbursement per resident is based on a historical figure set in 1996. Training has drastically changed since then, costing more money in educational tools such as simulation and seminar training, as well as faculty costs. Because of these changes, many of the hospitals are getting far less money than they are spending for each resident.

It is important to understand that YOU do not have funding that follows you, like a scholarship would. This funding is to subsidize the costs that the hospital has for being a teaching institution and employing a set number of residents that take care of Medicare and Medicaid patients. The hospital must track the location and training itineraries for all residents and fellows in order to determine which time can be claimed and which cannot be claimed. There are too many rules for this reporting to explain it here. Generally, they cannot claim time that you are outside of the clinical environment or rotations where you are visiting other teaching institutions. They can claim time that you are caring for patients in hospital affiliated clinical areas. The reimbursement is dependent on your eligibility and type of training program. With the capped limitations and regulations on what can and cannot be counted being very complex, the institution is very interested in maximizing the federal funding they receive to offset the overhead costs of running training programs. Therefore, while you don't have a dedicated funding, you do add to their federal funding when you are eligible. They can claim your time at 100% while you are eligible and only at 50% when you are past eligibility or in fellowship.

The number of years that you are eligible for this funding is directly determined by your "initial residency program." Whichever program you choose to join as a PGY1 will be your initial residency program, unless you participate in a transitional year where it is the PGY2 year that determines eligibility. The length of training that is designated for the initial residency program sets your eligibility for funding. If you begin in a surgical program, you will have five years. If you begin in family medicine, you will have three years. This will only matter to you if you choose to transfer to a different specialty, after you begin residency training. Let's consider examples to better explain the point.

Case #1 – Dr. Amy

Dr. Amy is interested in general surgery (GS), but she is also considering emergency medicine (EM). She matches into a five-year general surgery program. She spends two years in surgery and decides she wants to change to EM. The program directors for both GS and EM say she can transfer. What does she need to do?

If this is at the same institution, she needs to talk to her Designated Institutional Official (DIO) or Director of Medical Education. While the program directors may be fine with her transferring, there may be other issues that need to be addressed first. The DIO can assist Dr. Amy in determining if she can get any credit for her two years in surgery. The

DIO can determine if there are any eligibility issues with the transfer. The official transfer will require the DIO's approval. If Dr. Amy was going to another institution, both DIOs should be involved in the discussion.

In most cases, the resident that transfers will receive up to 6 months of credit in the new specialty, often called "advanced standing." Assuming this is the case for Dr. Amy, her training would look this:

> PGY1 – general surgery (R1)
> PGY2 – general surgery (R2)
> PGY3 – emergency medicine (R1)
> PGY4 – emergency medicine (R2)
> PGY5 – emergency medicine (R3) - graduate mid-year

In this case, Dr. Amy still graduates within her initial residency period (5 years), so funding is not an issue. The institution should have no objections based on eligibility. In addition, if Dr. Amy received the entire 6 months of advanced standing for her surgery training, she could be able to graduate with only two and a half more years of EM training. This means she could graduate off-cycle from her peers six months early.

Case # 2 – Dr. Matt

Dr. Matt like Dr. Amy is interested in both general surgery (GS) and emergency medicine (EM). He matches into emergency medicine, which is a three-year program. He spends two years in EM and decides he really enjoys the procedure side of medicine and requests a transfer to general surgery with the hopes of someday being a trauma surgeon. The program directors for both GS and EM say he can transfer. What does he need to do?

As with Dr. Amy, he needs to speak with his DIO to discuss the option of transferring and get approval for such a move. In this case, the institution may not be supportive, because there is an eligibility issue. He has already used two years of his three-year eligibility. If the institution is over their funding cap, it may not be an issue, but regardless, it will cost the institution more money that they originally agreed to when Dr. Matt was recruited to the initial program. Dr. Matt's training (assuming 6 months of advanced standing) in the new specialty would look like this:

> PGY1 – emergency medicine (R1)
> PGY2 – emergency medicine (R2)
> PGY3 – general surgery (R1)
> PGY4 – general surgery (R2)
> PGY5 – general surgery (R3)
> PGY6 – general surgery (R4)
> PGY7 – general surgery (R5) - graduate mid-year

In this case, Dr Matt's funding eligibility runs out after his PGY3 year. The institution will only be able to claim 50% of his time from PGY4 to PGY7. This will be a significant loss of funding...easily over $200,000 in losses for the institution over four years. If Dr. Matt is a valued resident that the institution hopes to keep after graduation, this may be supported by the administration. However, in most institutions, residents will have a difficult time selling this type of transfer to the DIO and hospital administration. In addition, if Dr. Matt want to specialize in trauma surgery, he would have to do a fellowship after residency training.

I shared these sample cases in order to give you an understanding that your choice for your PGY1 training is extremely important. If you are equally considering two specialties that have different training lengths, I highly recommend that you match into the longer program, so your options are not limited later, should you change your mind.

Types of PGY1

The PGY1 year is often referred to as the internship or intern year. The term "intern" is antiquated, but some faculty and hospital staff

14

continue to use it. ACGME and the GME offices tend to call it the PGY1 year. There are three terms referring to types of PGY1 years that you may hear as you research program options. These are Categorical, Preliminary, and Transitional year. If you are on message boards meant for medical students, please be aware that those that answer questions on these boards may have very limited knowledge and are only answering based on their personal experience. In other words, consider everything you read on these boards as potentially true or a part truth. The PGY1 year requirements have changed considerably in the past few years. Any information from per-2017 is potentially incorrect today and can be misleading or harmful to your career.

The majority of those reading this book will enter a Categorical position. This is a position where you enter directly into the specialty with plans to continue into PGY2 year in same program. If you meet the annual requirements for promotion, you will be promoted to the next level in the program. This is the standard type of PGY1 year that most programs offer, and most specialties require.

Preliminary Year and Transitional Year are very similar and often mixed up with each other. A Preliminary Year PGY1 position is where you enter into a specialty specific PGY1 program with no commitment for future training in same program. A Preliminary year resident may have the same training as a Categorical year resident in the same program. The difference is that the Preliminary resident has a single year commitment in the specialty residency program. Some programs will bring in Preliminary residents to fill out the ranks and provide additional coverage for rotations. In rare occasions, a categorical resident drops out of the program and a preliminary resident can get a categorical PGY2 contract at the end of the year.

A Transitional Year PGY1 position is a general PGY1 year with rotations in a wide variety of areas. This year is designed to give a broad range of experience to create a foundation for the PGY2 to build upon. It is also a single year commitment. Residents often match into a transitional year and their PGY2 year at the same time, so they have a commitment for their next year in a specialty program. The primary difference between preliminary and transitional positions is the specialized versus broad-based approach to the curriculum and experience. The transitional position will also be in an official Transitional Year (TY) Program, whereas the preliminary position is a track within the specialty residency program. There are several specialties that require either a preliminary year or Transitional year: Anesthesiology, Dermatology, Diagnostic Radiology, Nuclear Medicine, Ophthalmology, Osteopathic Neuromusculoskeletal Medicine, Physician Medicine and Rehabilitation, Preventive Medicine, and Radiation Oncology. At times a program can offer these PGY1 years at their institutions without having to match separately. For example, I know Anesthesiology and Physical Medicine & Rehabilitation programs that match PGY1s into a categorical position and provide the necessary training to move into the PGY2 position. When you decide on your specialty, make sure you have conversations with the GME offices at your preferred institutions. They will guide you on which positions to apply for, in order to enter your program of choice. Just remember that if you are applying for a PGY2 categorical position, you must have a PGY1 position as a prerequisite. Make sure you are applying for a PGY1 position as well.

There are some specialties that allow for multiple pathways. One example is Osteopathic Neuromusculoskeletal Medicine (ONM). You can do a Transitional Year (broad-based) as a foundation year of training, then enter the ONM residency for another two years. However, you can also do a three-year Family Medicine residency and add a single year of ONM as a fourth year. Both options allow you to be board eligible for ONM. However, when you do the Family Medicine pathway with the additional year of training, you can be both FM and ONM board eligible. This pathway is often referred to as a Plus One program. This provides you with more options for your career later. Table 3 is a comprehensive list of programs that currently require preliminary or transitional years. In some cases, institutions will be able to offer this PGY1 training and the residency training in the same location and with the same program.

Table 3: Programs that require Preliminary or Transitional Years

PGY 1	PGY 2	PGY 3	PGY 4	PGY 5
Preliminary Year	Anesthesiology			
Preliminary Year or Transitional Year	Dermatology			
Preliminary Year or Transitional Year	Diagnostic Radiology			
Preliminary Year or Transitional Year	Nuclear Medicine			
Preliminary year	Ophthalmology			
Transitional Year	Osteopathic Neuromusculoskeletal Medicine (ONM)			
Family Medicine			ONM	
Transitional Year	Physical Medicine and Rehabilitation			
Preliminary Year or Transitional Year	Preventive Medicine			
Preliminary Year or Transitional Year	Radiation Oncology			

The important concept to comprehend is that you need to understand the pathway to take in order to get to the board eligibility that you wish to pursue. There may be multiple options for your specialty or sub-specialty. Know your options and make sure to discuss with the programs how to appropriately apply for the relevant positions at those institutions.

So how do I choose?

Before you can decide on a specialty, you must know yourself, what type of environment you will excel in, and where you will not do well. Choosing a specialty is a journey that will take you a couple of years. Do not rush into anything and make sure that you leave your options open until you must decide. Give yourself plenty of time to experience as many of your potential choices as possible.

How do you experience your potential choices? Ask questions from different physicians as you have opportunities. Attend events that your school provides and join interest groups to explore your options further. If you have the opportunity to shadow physicians while on break, take the opportunity, even if it is for a couple of hours. Once you have clinical rotations, use your electives wisely. If you are interested in the surgical environment, rotate in Anesthesiology, General Surgery, Obstetrics, Orthopedics, etc. Get yourself into the operating room in as many rotations as you can. With this experience, you will truly get a chance to determine if this is the environment for you. The same advice goes for the in-patient or ambulatory environments. Choose as many rotations as you can to experience the environment, then consider each of the specialties that are in that environment.

Keep a journal of your experiences on all your rotations in your third year and fourth year. As you journal, pay attention to your feelings while on rotation. Were there rotations where you felt on point and at the top of your game? Were there rotations where you were uncomfortable or just not interested? Did you enjoy the form of communication and patient care that occurred on this rotation? Watch your attendings for clues about the lifestyle. What was the typical day for the attendings in this specialty? Talk to the residents and attendings about their choice of specialty. Journal your thoughts about your patient experiences. Free write in your journal at least once a week about your experience on the rotation. Before you pick your specialty, review all your journal entries. Are there any obvious winning specialties that stand out? The odds are that there will be definite negative experiences or feelings that will lead you away from a few specialties too. The importance of journaling is that we tend to remember the most recent experiences more than the ones we had a while ago. The journal will remind you of experiences that you may have forgotten. You should review it all, the good and the bad.

Time for self-reflection – Keep a Journal on your rotations

Now, that you have narrowed your search down based on your feelings and experiences, it is time to consider the option analytically. Here are some items that I recommend that you review and consider based on your own preferences. If you cannot answer these questions for the specialty that you are considering, find the answers. Talk to residents and attending physicians that you work with to figure out the answers and then determine if that is what you are really looking for in a career.

Things to consider when choosing your specialty:

- *Lifestyle* - What is the work-life balance in this specialty? Are you married to your work, or do you have time for family and personal hobbies? What work-life balance are you looking for? What work-life balance will you want in 10 year, 20 years, or 30 years? Is this a specialty that drains the life out of you? If so, you need to determine how you will maintain your own balance and personal wellness during training and later.

- *Length of training* – How many years will you have to train for this specialty, including residency and fellowships? Are you willing to put in the work for that number of years? Is the final lifestyle and salary worth the investment?

- *Work hours/shift time* – What is the typical day schedule? If it is an early morning, are you a morning person? Do you like working nights? Will you have to take call? Is the call in-house or from home? Would you work Monday through Friday or weekends too? Do you do a set number of shifts for the month, then take multiple days off? How many hours a week would you work on average?

- *USMLE and COMLEX-USA scores* – What are the expected scores for the specialty? Are you a competitive candidate? If you have borderline scores, you may want to consider something else. Generally, the longer programs have higher expectations for academic rigor. If you struggle with your board examination scores, you need to be realistic on your chances of getting into a competitive residency.

Picking the Right Specialty

- *Research requirements* – Some residency specialties have very intensive research requirements. For example, emergency medicine and general surgery expect you to be doing research that adds to the specialties' knowledge. You need to be publishing your research and presenting nationally during your residency training. What is your capability and/or interest level in doing this type of research during training and afterwards?

- *Physical requirements* – Do you have any physical limitations that need to be considered? Can you be on your feet for 8 hours hunched over an operating table? Can you run to a code, sometimes taking many flights of stairs? Make sure that you understand the physical needs of the specialty and whether you can meet those needs now and for decades into the future.

- *Communication style* – What is your communication style, and does it match the specialty that you are considering? Do you like to create a long-standing relationship with your patients such as family medicine? Would you prefer to diagnose and stabilize patients with limited follow up interaction like in emergency medicine? Are you interested in working with very sick patients and their family members? Do you want to practice medicine without seeing patients directly, such as radiology? Every specialty requires a specific type of communicator in order to be successful. Ask questions and learn about the communication skills you will need to thrive in your specialty.

- *Patient mix* - Do you have a specific demographic of patients with which you would like to work? If you enjoy working with children, you could consider family medicine and pediatrics, but you can also specialize in in pediatric subspecialties. Do you prefer adults? What about adults in pain or older adults?

- *Acuity of illness* – What type of illness acuity would you deal with in your chosen specialties? Do you have the intestinal fortitude to be surrounded by life threatening situations every day? Do you prefer working with severely ill patients or more mild conditions?

- *Preferred work environment* – Which setting would you prefer to work in - inpatient, outpatient, operating room, a dark radiology reading room, counseling office, etc. Do you want to work at the bedside or behind the scenes? Do you prefer the clinic, hospital, or surgery center environment?

Chapter Three:
Considering Your Program Options

Residency Programs

Now that you have determined your specialty or at least have it narrowed down considerably, you need to be strategic in selecting your elective rotations and using these to your advantage. Check with your school to see if you can rotate into hospitals where you wish to apply for the residency program. This type of rotation is called an "audition rotation." Some schools limit your rotations to within their own network of hospitals. If this is the case, it will be more difficult to audition outside of the network, but it is not impossible. You can still shadow during your break if need be. The important concept here is to use every opportunity to get in front of the right people to get their attention in a positive way.

Use every opportunity to get in front of the RIGHT people
to get their attention in a POSITIVE way

Before you determine where you want to do your elective rotations, you should determine where there are programs in the specialty that you are choosing. In addition, most medical students have a specific location or region in mind when they are applying for residency. Often the preferred location is near family for the benefit of a support system or in an area the student wishes to practice after residency. At times, the choice is where the best training is located, regardless of anything else. I have seen a few students move across the country just to get away from family for a while, then move back after residency. If you plan to have children during residency, you may have a higher need to be near extended family than if you are single without children. This is a very personal decision.

Once you have a specialty and geographic area in mind, you can go to the ACGME website to pull a list of all programs in that area for that specialty. You can then review those program websites for more information. The American Medical Association also maintains a database of programs called FREIDA. You can find more information about the program on the FREIDA website (https://freida.ama-assn.org/Freida/#/). This database provides a consistent formatting for the information on each program. Note that this is a sponsored advertisement database, not all programs pay for the expanded listing in the FREIDA database, but all programs will be listed with basic information at a minimum.

Once you know where the programs are, you need to determine the differences between the programs and which programs you wish to consider for yourself. Are you interested in a larger program or a smaller one? Would you like a university hospital or a community hospital? Some programs offer exposure to both settings. Are you interested in working in a rural area during residency or afterwards? There are programs with rural satellite options too. Look at the program websites for clues on the structure and environment of the program. Table 4 has a list of program characteristics that you may wish to consider. I suggest that you take this list and prioritize it for your own interests. Use this as an analysis tool when you are considering programs now and when you are finalizing your rank order list.

If you want to learn more about specific programs and can rotate at that institution, do so. When you apply for an audition rotation, you must be flexible with your dates. The more popular programs will have the schedule filled up very quickly. Audition rotations usually occur between August and December. This is a very busy time of year for the programs. At times, institutions will allow more students to rotate than they normally would during non-recruiting months, just to allow as many candidates as possible to visit the program. Therefore, if you are three students deep in the OR, do not be upset by this. Since you are there, that means that there are many more students that are not there in your place. These audition rotations are less about the curriculum and more about being seen. These rotations are about showing off your skills as a hard worker, quick learner, and the right "fit" for the program.

Make sure to schedule your audition rotations way in advance. If you are applying for a competitive program, you should be contacting them 6-9 months before you want to come. This means that if you want to rotate in the fall of your fourth year, you should schedule it in the middle of your third year. Do not wait until the end of year three to set up your fourth-year electives for August-December. Institutions will have an application process that you must use to schedule these rotations. Details are usually on the Medical Education websites for the institution.

You want to do audition rotations in August through December of your fourth year. You should be applying for these rotations in December through April of your third year.

Also, make sure you rotate in September or October at your assumed highest ranked programs. Why? Because, you may be forgotten if you rotate early in the season and you may be already written off if you rotate too late. Many programs will determine their favorites well before the December rotators begin. This does not mean you can't rotate in December. It just means that they will have favorite candidates that you will be compared to when you rotate. You will not be setting the standard; you will be defined by the standard that others have already set.

Considering Your Program Options

If your school limits your rotations, there are tricks to still get in front of the program. If you can only do one or two general surgery rotations and have already rotated in other places, you can still rotate in anesthesiology or another surgical specialty. You will still get into the operating room and potentially into other areas with the faculty from the program. Make your interests known. If you are well liked on that rotation, they will make sure you get to meet the program leadership and will recommend you to the program. This type of conversation about you is ideal.

Remember that whenever you are rotating clinically, you are interviewing for residency. Whether it is for those that will write letters for you or for those that will hire you. This is your opportunity to showcase your skills and abilities. Make sure that you have a strong work ethic throughout the entire rotation. This is very important for all rotations, not just the audition ones.

Another thing to remember is that everyone has the opportunity of helping you or hurting you. If they like you, you will be ranked higher than applicants that did not rotate, because they know you better than someone they interviewed, but that did not rotate with them. This is a double-edged sword, because if you are seen as a slacker or someone thinks negatively about you, you may go unranked. There is no rule that says the program must tell you if you are being ranked or not. They can choose to not rank you and not tell you. So be careful while on rotation at a facility that you wish to apply. Always put your best effort forward and watch your professionalism. The importance of this cannot be overstated. The attending physicians drive medical education. There is no room for error or bad behavior while in training.

When clinically rotating, always put your best effort forward
and watch your professionalism.

A common error that students make is to apply to two specialties in the same institution. The program administrators talk about their applicants and ask others in the institution about their experience while the student was rotating. If two programs both know you are applying, they will rightfully assume that you are not dedicated to their specialty. This could reduce your ranking on their match list. All programs want applicants that are excited to learn their specialty and dedicated to that specialty only. You can still apply for multiple specialties; I recommend that you do not do this is the same institution for the reason above.

Fellowship Programs

All ACGME accredited fellowship programs are related to specific residency programs through their accreditation. In this relationship, the residency program is called the parent program to the fellowship. The parent program's director is responsible for oversight of the fellowships that are connected to the residency program. Consider the fellowship programs as extensions of the residency programs. In reality, the residency program director works together with the fellowship program directors to ensure that all programs are meeting accreditation requirements.

Like residency programs, it is very common for fellowships to choose residents that they know, over unknown candidates. If you have an interest in a fellowship program, it is highly recommended that you consider applying for the parent residency program. You are not guaranteed a fellowship position if you attend the parent residency program. However, it puts you at a better advantage then those that did not go to the parent residency. If the parent residency is not of interest to you, do a little research to see what other programs the previous fellows have graduated from. Program directors tend to trust programs that they have had good experiences with and often will consider graduates from those programs more favorably than others. Those are the programs that you want to consider applying to, if you are determined to get into this specific fellowship.

Considering Your Program Options

Table 4: Program Characteristics

PROGRAM CHARACTERISTICS TO CONSIDER:	
• Accreditation status & history • Number of faculty • Quality of faculty • Size of program • Mentorship program • Performance feedback from faculty • Supervision and participation of faculty at night • Salary rate • Non-salary benefits (examples: food, educational stipend, fringe benefits, etc.) • Moonlighting opportunities • Sponsoring institution facilities • Sponsoring institution location • GME department and resident relationships • Residency program director and leadership • Diversity of geographic location • Diversity of sponsoring institution	• Quality of didactic sessions • Quality of bedside teaching • Patient mix, scope, and volume • Opportunity for patient continuity of care • Quality of ambulatory experience • Night call schedule • Rotational experience • Elective opportunities • Research curriculum • Quality of Research Projects • Quantity of Research Publications • Current resident satisfaction with program • Reputation of the program • Reputation of the hospital • Use of technology • Board pass rates • Community connection • Cost of living • Future opportunities after graduation

Osteopathic Recognition

Another program characteristic that we have not discussed is Osteopathic Recognition. This is an ACGME program recognition, in addition to the specialty accreditation, which indicates that the program has been recognized for its commitment to teaching and assessing Osteopathic Principles and Practice (OPP). These programs are open to all medical students. You do not need to be a graduate of an Osteopathic medical school and not all residents in an Osteopathic Recognized program need to participate in the OPP training. So, what is OPP?

To understand Osteopathic Principles and Practice and the Osteopathic philosophy, we need to know about Andrew Taylor Still. Dr. Still was a typical frontier physician who became a physician officer during the Civil War.[1] After his war experience and the death of several family members to spinal meningitis and pneumonia, Dr. Still began questioning traditional medicine and searching for better methods to treat his patients. His work was based on the structural relationship between bones, muscles, and organs. Before long, he became known as a magnetic healer that provided drugless, manipulative medicine.

In 1885, Dr. Still's version of medicine was officially named "Osteopathy." When he had more patients that he could personally treat, he decided to open the American School of Osteopathy (ASO) in 1892. In 1895, more than 30,000 osteopathic treatments occurred in the ASO Infirmary. It is estimated that 400 patients came to Kirksville, Missouri each day for treatment. Railroad schedules were changed to accommodate the inflex of people visiting ASO, now called A.T. Still University (ATSU). ATSU was the first Osteopathic medical school. Today, the American Osteopathic Association (AOA) oversees all Osteopathic training and board certification. Currently, the AOA's

---

[1] A.T. Still University, *A.T. Still Biography* (2019). Retrieved at:
https://www.atsu.edu/museum-of-osteopathic-medicine/museum-at-still.

Commission on Osteopathic College Accreditation has 38 accredited osteopathic medical schools with 59 locations in the USA.[2] This accounts for approximately 25% of all USA medical students. There are more than 145,000 Doctors of Osteopathy (D.O.) practicing medicine today.

The American Osteopathic Association has identified four underlying Tenets for the philosophy of osteopathic medicine:

- The person is a unit of body, mind, and spirit.
- The body is capable of self-regulation, self-healing, and health maintenance.
- Structure and function are reciprocally interrelated.
- Rational treatment is based upon an understanding of the basic principles of body unity, self-regulation, and the interrelationship of structure and function.

These Tenets are part of the OPP training taught to all Osteopathic medical students and residents. In 2014, the ACGME and AOA announced a five-year plan to transition all AOA residency programs to ACGME. By July 2020, the AOA is no longer accrediting residency programs.

With this transition, the ACGME has created Osteopathic Recognition (OR) to officially identify those programs that wish to continue the Osteopathic Principles and Practices which Dr. Still began over a century ago. Osteopathic Recognition requires a minimum of one resident per class level to participate in the OPP training. More than one can participate in the training, but only one is required to continue the program's OR status. Therefore, in a program which has Osteopathic Recognition, all residents may participate in OPP or part of the residents may participate in OPP. This has allowed some previously Osteopathic (AOA) residency programs to continue with their traditional training of

---

2   American Osteopathic Association (2019). *Osteopathic Medical Schools*. Retrieved at: https://osteopathic.org/about/affiliated-organizations/osteopathic-medical-schools/

OPP. It has also allowed some historically non-Osteopathic programs to incorporate new OPP curricula to expand the training of their residents.

There is no universal requirement or minimum standard for eligibility to participate in Osteopathic Recognition residency positions. The programs can determine their own pre-requisite requirements. Osteopathic medical schools should automatically meet the qualification requirements based on the curriculum that is required for medical school graduation. Allopathic medical school graduates or those that never received Osteopathic training may be required to participate in workshops or special training in order to satisfy pre-requisite requirements in Osteopathic training, as determined by their residency program.

If you are considering programs with Osteopathic Recognition, make sure that you ask how they are filling the OR positions. Are all positions expected to participate in the OPP curriculum? Can residents pick if they are interested in an OR position after the Match? Osteopathic Recognition can be beneficial training for your future career. It is worth considering, whether you are an Osteopathic student or not. You can find out more information about Osteopathic Recognition at the ACGME website.[3]

---

[3] Accreditation Council for Graduate Medical Education (2019). *Osteopathic Recognition*. Retrieved from: https://www.acgme.org/What-We-Do/Recognition/Osteopathic-Recognition.

Chapter Four:
Preparing the ERAS application

Before you begin the application process, you need to understand the process and prepare accordingly. As we already discussed, knowing the specialty and potential residency programs you are interested in applying to is very important. Your school will inform you of the detailed process of submitting your applications. However, you need to make sure that you spend the necessary time in preparation to be successful in your pursuits.

Your application will contain your academic record, scholarly activity, personal statement, letters of reference, and community involvement. Each selection committee will have their own expectations for candidates. However, each specialty has standards that are somewhat universal across the programs. For example, if you wish to enter a competitive specialty such as orthopaedic surgery, you will be expected to have a robust list of research or publications listed on your application. For many less competitive programs, as a minimum, you should have participated in research day presentations as a medical student.

You should determine if the programs have specific requirements for selection. Every program is required to have a selection policy. You may be able to find this information on their program website. While some programs will advertise cut off scores for USMLE or COMLEX-USA, many others do not publicly provide such information. You may need to access this information through discussions with the program director or program coordinator.

Be Realistic

Up to this point, we have discussed your specialty interests. Now it is time to be realistic and discuss what specialties you qualify for given your academic background. A great resource to help you be realistic is to look at the National Residency Match Program's (NRMP) "Interactive Charting Outcomes in the Match" website.[4] There is a separate interactive website link for USMLE and COMLEX-USA data where average scores are identified by specialty. Each year, the NRMP also publishes a report with this data that can be downloaded in PDF format. Review this data to determine the historical expectations within your preferred specialty. Is your Step I or Level I score at or above last year's average for your preferred specialty? If the answer to this question is no, you may need to rethink your specialty options.

Let's look at an example of these data points. The PDF report called NRMP Charting Outcomes in the Match 2018 indicates that the most competitive residency programs based on USMLE score are Dermatology, Interventional Radiology, Neurological Surgery, Orthopaedic Surgery, Otolaryngology, Plastic Surgery, and Radiation Oncology.[5] Those that matched in these specialties had an average Step I score of 245 or higher. In contrast, family medicine had an average score of 218 and Physical Medicine and Rehabilitation had an average score around 222. These charts can help you determine what specialties are reasonable with your current transcript of scores. This same report also indicates that those that do not match in these specialties have lower scores than those that matched. There are more data points, such as work experience, research

---

[4] National Matching Residency Program (2019). *Interactive Charting Outcomes in the Match*. Retrieved from: http://www.nrmp.org/interactive-charting-outcomes-in-the-match/

[5] National Matching Residency Program (2018). *Charting Outcomes in the Match: U.S. Allopathic Seniors, 2018*, p. 9. Retrieved from: https://www.nrmp.org/wp-content/uploads/2018/06/Charting-Outcomes-in-the-Match-2018-Seniors.pdf

experience, presentations, volunteer experience, etc. I highly recommend that you review these reports to determine if you are a quality candidate for the specialty that you prefer.

Another NRMP report that may be of interest to you is the annual NRMP Applicant Survey by Preferred Specialty and Applicant Type.[6] This survey gives you information about the most recent match and how medical students ranked the importance of program data for making decisions, how many programs they interviewed with, how many programs they applied to, how many went through the SOAP, etc. This report may provide some insight into your specialty choice and help you develop a strategic plan to be matched.

Complete Application

Each program will have an expectation for what constitutes a complete application. Many programs will not review your application until it is complete. Make sure that you have the following included in your application:

- Three letters of reference
- Examination transcript
- Curriculum Vitae with scholarly activity
- Medical School Performance Evaluation (Dean's Letter)
- Medical school transcript
- Professional photo
- Personal statement

---

[6] National Matching Residency Program (2019). *Results of the 2019 NRMP Applicant Survey by Preferred Specialty and Applicant Type.* Retrieved from: https://mk0nrmp3oyqui6wqfm.kinstacdn.com/wp-content/uploads/2019/06/Applicant-Survey-Report-2019.pdf.

Letters of Reference

A program will look at the number of Letters of Reference you have in your file and may not review it until you have their specific requested number. Most programs look for three letters. Program directors and faculty like to review letters written by physicians that you have worked with. It is very important that you have at least three flattering letters from physicians, preferably in the field you wish to pursue.

The application system allows letters to be submitted without your review. If you choose this option, make sure you are very comfortable that the person writing the letter is very supportive of you. Programs read hundreds of letters each recruitment session. They are very good at recognizing slight differences in letters that can say a lot about the candidate. Letters that state that they worked with you on a rotation and you were on time and professional are great. Compare that to a letter that states you were striving to increase your knowledge throughout by reading ahead and asking excellent questions. The better the writer knows you and the longer they worked with you the better the Letter of Reference. If you worked on a research project with a faculty member, make sure they write you a letter. This type of letter is always helpful, assuming you did a great job on the project and took the project seriously, maybe even did a presentation with the data.

It is very important that you have at least three flattering letters from physicians, preferably in the field you wish to pursue.

If you are applying in multiple specialties, you will need to have two separate applications filled out. This way you can ensure that the letters and personal statement are identifying the correct specialty. Placing a personal statement, about your lifelong dream of being a surgeon, in your emergency medicine application will be an automatic red flag that you are not the candidate for them. Make sure that everything is specific to the specialty that you are attempting to enter with that specific application.

Examination transcript

You will need to have your USMLE or COMLEX-USA transcripts attached to your application. When you have updates to your examination scores, make sure new transcripts are posted. Some programs will interview you with only your Level I/Step I transcripts. However, it is common practice not to rank a candidate without seeing passing Level II/Step II transcripts in the application. You may wonder why this is the case. In order to graduate from medical school and/or get a training license, you need to be successful in your Level II/Step II examination. Programs that Rank candidates without seeing this passing score have historically been hurt when candidates were unsuccessful in passing Level II/Step II before the residency start date. This has led to matched medical students being released from their matched programs and positions going unfilled. To eliminate this potential problem, many institutions have set rules that candidates must have passed both levels of their examinations in order to be ranked.

It is common practice not to rank a candidate without seeing passing Level II/Step II transcripts in the application.

You need to take the USMLE and COMLEX USA examinations very seriously. While you can retake them should you fail, a single failing score on your transcript can negatively impact your candidacy. Some programs overlook the previous fail, if you have an explanation in your personal statement that shows it was a one-time issue. An example of this type of explanation may be that you had a family member pass away or you became very ill just prior to the examination. If your second attempt shows an excellent score, this would support the explanation. If your second attempt is a low passing score, you will not be able to explain away your first failing score. Having only passing scores on your transcript is so important that some schools have created policies to keep students from taking the examinations until they have proven that they are ready.

Curriculum Vitae with Scholarly Activity

While the Curriculum Vitae (CV) is optional on ERAS, I recommend that you have one submitted. Your CV is a running list of your education, accomplishments, and scholarly activity. It is a great tool for the program to review your career pathway and special skills. A good CV will have the following information:

- Name and contact information
- Education
- Certifications
- Employment
- Scholarly activity
- Associations
- Community Involvement

Use the CV to show your unique qualifications and to provide more information on the projects you have been involved with throughout your educational pursuits. List your research projects, specialty interest groups, student government, volunteer work, etc. The format is not as important as the data on the CV. Your CV should not include a photo or any personal information such on your date of birth or marital status. You may see CVs of mature physicians with this information, but it is a not the current expectation of a professional CV.

Make sure that you develop a CV in a Word document that you can easily add to as the years go on. Do not use tables or fancy formatting, as it may not translate well when you distribute the file. Every presentation or project should be listed on this CV. Every certification or specialized training that you participate in should be noted as well. It is your career blueprint. Create a CV for your application and update it at least annually throughout your residency. You will be grateful that you did.

Use the CV to show your unique qualifications
and to provide more information on the projects

Medical School Performance Evaluation (Dean's Letter)

Medical School Performance Evaluation (MSPE), often referred to as the Dean's Letter, is your school's review of your training. It is a standardized letter that the school creates for each student. Each school provides a narrative about your training and how you performed in relation to your peers. Some schools provide this information in the format of a letter of reference. Other schools provide specific comments from your faculty that were solicited throughout your training. This letter, along with your medical school transcript, provides the programs with insight on your academic rigor in a formal setting. Some programs will not send out interview offers until they have reviewed the MSPE. Other programs do not wait for the MPSE to invite applicants, but use it to support their ranking decisions after you have interviewed.

Medical School Transcript

Your transcript will include your course work and final grades. Some medical schools use a pass and fail grading system, so it is difficult for the programs to use the transcript to rank your candidacy. Therefore, the programs tend to review the transcript for red flags only. If you passed every class and rotation, the transcript should not affect your candidacy. Those that have had failures or have had to retake classes or rotations will be considered a bit more closely. If you were delayed from graduating on time, due to an academic issue, you may be considered a risky candidate for the program. If you have any red flags on your transcript, you MUST address them in your personal statement. If you do not, you may never get the opportunity to explain yourself.

Professional photo

If your school does not offer a photography shoot, you should set up a shoot with a professional photographer yourself. Go for a very simple background and have a headshot taken. Be professionally dressed and smile. Refer to my biography photo for an example. A good photo will be helpful for years. You can use it for scholarly activity events in the future as well. In addition, you should add it to your professional social media profile, such as LinkedIn.

You may ask why you need a photo on your application. Many institutions and/or programs do not use the photo in the interview selection process. ERAS has an option for institutions to block out photos and demographic information. This option is often used to ensure non-discriminatory practices throughout the institution's programs. However, often the photo is used to identify you on interview day, in ranking discussions, and may be used in welcome announcements. In addition, you will likely have a formal photo taken in your lab coat at orientation. This will be used by your hospital to identify you to other staff using welcome flyers and maybe an online GME profile, etc.

Personal statement

Writing your Personal Statement is time consuming and exhausting. I could write an entire book on the subject and plan to someday. What you need to know to get started is that your personal statement is your personal movie trailer for your residency candidacy. This is your chance to tell them, in one or two pages, why you are the student they want to hire. It should be a clearly written cohesive life story leading to your medical specialty and career interests. It should not be boastful listing of your accomplishments or a reiteration of your CV.

Preparing the ERAS Application

In your personal statement, you can go in several different directions. You can highlight what makes you a unique candidate, you can give the story behind your specialty choice, or you can expound upon the future and discuss your future goals. The best statements are creative and give a look into your personality, in other words it is "personal."

Here are some questions to ask yourself while preparing to write your personal statement:

- What makes you unique?
    - What strengths, skills, and experience will you bring to this specialty?
    - What motivates you?
    - What makes you a good fit for the specialty?
    - Why did you choose this specialty?
    - Do you have a story to tell?
    - Did you have a special skill to highlight?
    - Is this a second career for you?
- What appeals to you about the specialty?
    - How did you make your choice?
    - What are your current career goals?
- Do you have red flags to explain?
    - Did you fail an examination or rotation?
    - Where you delayed in graduating for any reason?

I would encourage you to take a few weeks to write your statement. Start by doing a draft using a "free writing" process. Just get some ideas down on paper and set it aside for 1-2 days. Then review your first draft, crossing out less important thoughts and circle the main thoughts that you want to bring forward, add anything else that comes to mind. Set it aside for 1-2 days. It will take you about four to five drafts to get something that you may consider using. Then, have at least two peers review for content, grammar, and typographical errors.

Preparing the ERAS Application

Here are some tips for writing a personal statement:

- **Do:**
  - Focus on the specialty.
  - Consider customizing by type of program (large vs small, research vs clinical, community hospital vs university based).
  - Share a patient encounter or story of interest that led you to your specialty choice.
  - Show insight and maturity of thought.
  - Be honest.
  - Keep your non-medical extracurricular activities out of the statement, unless they are pertinent to the story.
  - Use a tone and style that will sell your accomplishments without being arrogant or boastful.
  - Show, rather than tell about, your strengths using examples within your story.
  - Begin with an intriguing paragraph about your past, i.e. quote a mentor or patient.
  - Use suspense to arouse curiosity.
  - Start with the story and end with the conclusion.
  - Use irony and contrasting only when appropriate.
  - Open with a failure and discuss how you changed a failure to a success.
  - Talk about a mentor that influenced your choice in specialty and highlight ways you may be different.

- **Don't:**
    - Rehash your Curriculum Vita.
    - Use famous quotes unless you can really work the entire statement around them. The poor use of quotes is distracting to the reader.
    - Include information on your marital status, age, race, or religion.
    - Use humor or statements that can be interpreted as immature or goofy.
    - Use jargon or slang, unless in a quote for your story.

How to stand out from the crowd

If you are reading this book, you have already shown your interest in being proactive in developing your career. The best way of proactively standing out in the crowd is to develop your scholarly activity during medical school. If you haven't already done so, get involved in scholarly activity NOW! So what does that mean? Scholarly activity is a vague term which means that you are actively engaged in scholarly pursuits. Most scholarly pursuits will lead to the presentation of your project at a conference, research forum, or in a publication. Depending on your specialty, you may be expected to have a publication during medical school or at least while in residency. Not all projects are publishable or even presentable at conferences. Some of your projects may be community-based initiatives or Quality Improvement (QI) projects where only a small group of people may be interested in the results. Regardless of the presentation type, you need to make sure that you are tracking all projects that may be considered scholarly activity. Take credit for your work in your CV and application. If you have helped to develop a better clinical process with a mentor, claim the project. If you worked on providing improved care to a specific group of people while working on a resident's QI project, claim the project. The idea here is to show that you have the skills and knowledge to participate now and, in the future, to develop and lead projects that can make a difference in the lives of others. Scholarly activity in some specialties is identified as giving back to the field by publishing new information or suggestions for improvement within the specialty. At a minimum, investigate medical student competitions where you can present a poster, such as a community research forum or medical school research forum. Reach out to a mentor or resident that you respect and ask if you can help with their projects. They often need students to do chart reviews or literature searches. Get involved and take the opportunity to learn.

Managing Your Social Media and Cameras

Long before you are applying for residency programs, you need to rethink your use of social media. Potential employers and residency programs can and will search for you on the web. You want your online presence to be professional and uncomplicated. Patients will also search for your name. You need to guard yourself from patients that are too intrusive, but also you need to make patients feel comfortable with you as their physician.

The presence of unprofessional material on your social media can limit your career opportunities and cause complications with patients. Each institution and program will have their own expectations for their candidates. Some institutions may have stricter expectations, such as faith-based organizations. Before you apply to residency, you should ensure that your social media accounts are PG-rated and non-political. You need to look at your posts with a new set of eyes. If you have pictures that show you drinking with friends, you don't have to remove them. Just make sure they are mature and appropriate for a physician. The presence of alcohol alone is not a problem. You can have a photo of you enjoying a bottle of wine with your colleagues at a conference. You may not want to include the photos from your buddy's bachelor (or bachelorette) party though. You may want to reconsider the beach photos with scantily clad bikini bodies. Even if marijuana is legal in your state, do not share photos of you or anyone else using it. (Side note: Make sure you are not using it or you will not pass the pre-employment drug screen.)

Think of social media as being divided into professional accounts and personal accounts. The professional accounts are for colleagues, potential employers, faculty, and patients to see, such as LinkedIn. It is advisable to have a professional social media account to connect with others in your field. This account can be used to provide information in a professional manner and stay in touch with colleagues after you no longer work together or after you meet someone at a conference. This type of account can have your CV material in the profile but be careful not to include too personal of information. Remember, patients will be looking at this account as well. There will be a day when a patient is not happy with you or a patient's family member is seeking you out. Do not give them any information on your home location or any inappropriate posts that they can use against you.

Keep your professional and personal accounts separated and guard your personal accounts with high security settings.

Personal accounts are for your family and friends. It is helpful to change your personal social media account security to the highest security setting. Some social media profiles can be locked down to only show your photos and posts to your friends. Remember that your profile photo is usually seen by anyone that searches your name, so it needs to be professional looking regardless of your security settings. Personal accounts are not 100% protected when you use high security settings. Be aware that your "Friends" or connections on your personal account may use your posts against you in the future. Never share anything about your patients or the type of cases that you treated on social media. You may think it is just visible by your friends, but it can still be a HIPAA violation[7]. I have seen residents turn in other residents for posting too specific of information about their day. In my years of administration, I have seen several residents disciplined and even fired for inappropriate social medial posts. Remember, you are not the one that determines if it was a violation, the hospital administration makes that determination.

Camera Usage

You should never use your phone to take pictures at a clinical site or hospital unless it is approved by your institution in writing. Institutions have very strict rules about this. You may have seen students or residents post videos or pictures from a hospital setting. I have personally known residents that have been released from their programs because they misused their cameras in this manner.

Do not use your personal camera in a clinical setting
without prior authorization and understanding
the institution's policies regarding camera use.

We all know that you cannot take pictures of patients, but students often don't realize that they cannot take pictures of themselves or their peers on campus. Some institutions will limit use of cameras in

---

[7] U.S. Department of Health & Human Services (2019). Health Information Privacy, Retrieved from: https://www.hhs.gov/hipaa/for-professionals/index.html.

recognizable areas or by institutional signs, while others have a complete ban on the use of personal cameras. If you need to take a picture of a patient for a research poster, check with your GME office on policies regarding proper procedure. Some institutions require you to use a specific institutionally owned camera. Other institutions allow you to use your own camera, if you get a written release from the patient. Never assume that you can use your personal camera at a healthcare campus.

Chapter Five:
Communicating with Programs and Interviewing

Program Structure

In order to know how to communicate appropriately, you need to understand the organizational structure of a residency program. The residency program will have a program director (PD) and training administrator (TA). Large programs have two administrators and may have other support staff. The program may be located in a central GME office or may be in the specialty's clinical location. If it is in the GME office, you may have other GME staff that cross cover duties for the program. Some institutions have a dedicated staff member that communicates with all new residents for on-boarding purposes and/or recruiting logistics.

So, what is the training administrator's role in the program? The TA role has changed over the last 20 years and may be different from institution to institution. Programs use to have program secretaries. The program secretary used to be a secretary to the director that would maintain training records and type program communication. In 2001, there were significant changes to ACGME accreditation requirements. Around this time, many programs developed dedicated program coordinator roles to actively oversee residency documentation and assist the program director in meeting accreditation standards. The coordinator maintains program documentation for accreditation, tracks faculty/resident activity, maintains rotation schedules, etc. With additional accreditation requirements developed over the next decade, GME has become very complex. Program coordinators recognized that their role was changing and that a very specialized field was developing. In 2006, the role of a program coordinator was elevated with the creation of a professional certification, Training Administrator of Graduate Medical Education (TAGME). Fast forward to the present and you can see that the Training Administrator (TA) is a partner with the program director. The TA still does all the tasks of a PC, but also sits on committees, maintains milestones and goals & objectives, manages accreditation site visits, and ensures that the program maintains accreditation by advising the director and often acting on the director's behalf in communications and planning. This may mean the TA will mentor the residents on administrative responsibilities to ensure things are done on time. Each program may treat the TA position differently. Some programs will have a PC and a TA. Create a good relationship with the TA and it will be beneficial to you if/when you enter that residency program. Often the TA is seen as a less threatening program leader that you can go to with questions, special needs, and frustrations.

**The most successful physicians treat all people
with kindness and respect regardless of their role.**

Consider the TA as an extension of the program director. TAs are the gate keepers of the programs. Treat them with respect in every interaction. Trust them when they tell you the status of your application or that you need to do something. Often, the TA is the first reviewer of applications. They will verify that the application is complete and that it meets program minimum standards. The biggest mistake that medical students make is to treat the TA or GME staff poorly. The most successful physicians treat all people with kindness and respect regardless of their role. TAs are often partners in the ranking process with their opinions influencing the rank list or for some it is a veto power over difficult or needy candidates. TAs know that if candidates are difficult while they are courting the program, they will be far worse when they are matched. It is their job to identify the unprofessional and those that can't seem to follow directions.

Selection Process

Each program will have their own selection process. In general, once the TA reviews and forwards your application, a selection committee of faculty and/or senior residents will determine who will be offered an interview. Those identified for interview will be invited by the TA.

The TA will likely email the candidate with an invitation to interview on specific dates. The candidate will have a limited time to respond to the invitation. All communication tends to be done through the email system in the ERAS application. Interview dates fill up quickly, so do not delay long before responding to a program. The invitations are sent to more people than there are interview slots. Try to respond right away, but if you must hold off to determine your plans, respond within 2-3 days of receiving an invitation. If you wait too long to respond, your interview offer will become a place on the "waiting list" for an open interview timeslot. Most programs will offer a select number of interview dates. Some smaller programs will offer one or two dates, while bigger programs may offer up to ten dates. It is common for interviews to be on Thursday or Friday so you can travel home on the weekend.

When you interview, you will either meet individually with interviewers or you may be interviewed by a panel. Programs will often provide an introductory session where you can speak with the PD and ask questions. Tours of the facility are common. Some programs will schedule interview days along with didactic sessions or Grand Rounds, so you get a glimpse into the program. It is important to take advantage of these opportunities to see how the residents and faculty interact. Look for programs with camaraderie, but not too much. There should be a teacher-student relationship with positive reinforcement. If the faculty and residents are too close or familiar with each other's personal lives, it may signal a program with little boundary for personal space. This can lead to complexities during residency for those not comfortable with this type of program. Remember, the director and faculty are not your friends, the director is your boss and the faculty are your supervisors.

It is common to have a social event with all the candidates either the night before or night of the interviews. These events may be include going to a bar, restaurant, bowling alley, sporting event, etc. You should attend any events that are offered, if you can work your travel plans around these events. These events tend to be primarily with current residents, so you can get to know your potential peer group. Be very careful not to be pulled into the residents' web at these events. The residents may encourage you to relax and enjoy yourself. However, they are tasked with determining if you are a good fit for their program. There may be drinking, but you need to make sure you remain sober and appropriate in all your interactions. Some programs have prided themselves on having a "beer and chicken wings" culture. Others look to provide a higher-class experience to their candidates. Regardless of the event, do not get pulled into inappropriate conversations or rumors about others. Make sure you do not participate in sexual, discriminatory, or inappropriate humor. You never know what will happen when drinking is involved, and inhibitions are relaxed. I have seen several people removed from the Rank Order List due to the residents' not liking the candidates, the candidate drank in excess, or the candidate was inappropriate in some other way during the social event.

Remember that this social event is a test, so be prepared to pass the test. The test goes both ways, if you are uncomfortable with the interactions at this social event, it will be a big clue that this is not the program for you.

Communicating with Programs

After the interview day, it is advisable to send a thank you note to the interviewers. This is traditional etiquette, but not many people do it anymore. An email thank you is acceptable. If you do not have the interviewers' email addresses, you can send a combined email to the TA addressed to the program leadership and your interviewers. The TA will share with the director and others listed. This shows your continued interest in the program and that you know professional etiquette.

You may also wish to stay connected with some of the residents via email. You must follow the NRMP Match communication guidelines[8] with all program representatives, including residents, but a personal note to the residents reiterating your interest or following up on a conversation that you had earlier may be fruitful. It could also provide a connection for future scholarly activity, if nothing else.

After all the interviews are completed, you may receive an email from the PD or TA that states that you are being ranked. It is not common but may occur. The NRMP Match has very strict guidelines on how you communicate with the program and how they communicate with you about the Match. You can both volunteer that you are ranking each other, but you cannot ask each other how you are being ranked. If you receive any further communication, you can assume you are being ranked, unless it is specifically saying that you will not be ranked or is a benign email thanking you for your application.

If you do not get an interview invitation from a program by mid-November, you probably will not. It is common to send out invitations in September and October. If another interview date is set up, they may extend new invitations in November, but it is uncommon. The last possible interview dates would be early January. If you were not invited

---

[8] National Matching Residency Program (2019). *Match Participation Agreements*. Retrieved from: http://www.nrmp.org/match-participation-agreements/

to interview, you will not be ranked. Do not bother ranking those programs.

Communicating with the Programs

Most of your communication will be via email through the ERAS software. Make sure to check your email daily and respond quickly to the programs when they email you. It can be very expensive to interview at multiple institutions, if airfare and hotels are involved. Therefore, some programs can work you into an impromptu interview while you are rotating with them, so you do not have the additional expense of traveling back on a formal interview day. It does not hurt to ask. You will not be seen as cheap, rather as being efficient with your time and money.

If you have not heard from a program, it is okay to call the TA to inquire about your application. The program will never call you to tell you the application is not complete. You need to contact them to ensure that you meet their needs. Make sure that you are courteous and professional in your communication. They will look your application up in the ERAS system and provide you with an update. If you need more items, they can tell you at this point. If you have not been reviewed or have not been invited to interview, the TA may not tell you this. You may be told that your application is still under consideration. You can ask when the last interview invitations will be sent out. That way you will know after that date that you did not get an interview at this program. Some programs will send out a mass email to the candidates that were not invited to interview thanking them for their applications. Most do not communicate with you at all, if you are not invited to interview. Be aware that many programs are dealing with hundreds of applicants. You will have to request information from them, if they do not contact you for an interview.

What is professional communication?

There are times when you will communicate with the programs to ask for an audition rotation, request further information on their selection criteria, respond to interview requests, etc. At all times, know whom you are communicating with and address them accordingly when you send an email or make a phone call. Emails should be addressed "Dear Dr. ___" for program directors, "Dear Ms. or Mr. Last Name" for staff (unless they have a doctorate degree then "Dr."), or "To Whom It May Concern" if you need to be generic. If the staff member tells you to call him or her by their first name, you should still use the formal address in written communication. Your letters of reference should all be addressed "To Whom It May Concern." Make sure that physicians or doctorate level leadership are appropriately addressed as "Dr." Nothing shows disrespect more than using "Mr." because you did not take the time to look up the person's credentials.

Make sure that your language in your communication is proper English, without slang or informal phrasing. I have seen several candidates dismissed, because they acted like they were too familiar with the director in their writing. Remember, you are applying for a job and you need to act like you would if you were applying for a professional position anywhere.

If you inquire about your application with the TA, you may not like the response that you receive. Continuing to contact the TA multiple times about the same issue is not seen as being persistent, it is a red flag that you will be a difficult resident. You need to take the feedback provided to you and move along. Arguing with the TA about the quality of your application and why they did not choose you for interview will not get you an interview. It will, however, guarantee that you could be blacklisted at that institution and/or others associated with that institution.

You need to understand that there is no privacy expectation on the part of the programs. While programs do not share the full application with other programs, it is common for TAs in the same sponsoring institution to talk among themselves about good and bad candidates. If you get on their radar as a bad candidate, you will be the topic of conversation. The stories are routinely shared between the staff when there is a persistently bullying, unprofessional, or disrespectful candidate. Your name will get out there and you will have a reputation based on your communication techniques.

The good news is that a quality candidate with exceptionally professional communication will also be discussed and when you get a reputation for being respectful and professional, you have a higher chance of being ranked highly.

Things to Remember:
- There is a fine line between persistent and pest.
- Keep in touch with PD and/or residents after rotations.
- Treat EVERYONE with respect.
- The TA is the GATE KEEPER!
- Applications will not be considered until they are complete, and it is YOUR responsibility to ensure they are complete.
- **ALWAYS BE PROFESSIONAL!**

Gathering pertinent information

Before you began communicating with the programs, you reviewed their website and learned about their institutions. If you used the list found in Table 4 to review program characteristics, you probably already reviewed a large amount of data about each program. Hopefully, you have ranked this characteristics list from the most important to least important, so you can use it to guide your decisions now. When you are interviewing, take the opportunity to ask all the questions that you could not answer in your previous research about the program. Do not waste your time discussing information that is on the website, unless you want to independently verify information. The program will be happy to answer your questions and you will show that you have been thoughtful in your decision to interview with this program.

Determine which items to discuss with each group, then create a potential question list for your interview day. Examples may include:

- Ask the residents about their everyday experience, quality of teaching, availability of adequate supervision, case load, formal didactic instruction, wellness events, etc.
- Ask the faculty about their expectations for residents at each level in the program, how they determine the level of supervision they need to provide to each resident, their scholarly activity and special research interests, etc.
- Ask the director what he is looking for in a quality candidate, are there any planned changes to the curriculum for next year, number of projected out-rotations, expectations for scholarly activity, etc.
- Ask the TA any financial questions or about statistical data that shows the quality of the program…board pass rates, average in-training exam performance, active citations from the ACGME, etc.

If the program has been placed on a probationary status through the ACGME, the program is supposed to inform you of that status. Always know the accreditation status of the programs to which you are applying. If the program is in trouble and does not have a strategic plan to return to full accreditation, you may not wish to rank that program. Check ACGME.org for accreditation status.

The Interview

Before you begin interviewing, you need to determine your budget. Interviewing at multiple programs in different regions can be costly. Some programs will provide a hotel stipend or travel assistance, but this is not the norm and should not be expected. You should approach the interview season with the expectation that you will need to pay for all expenses to interview at 12-15 programs. In 2019, US Allopathic Senior NRMP applicants who matched were invited to interview at an average of 17 programs and chose to interview at 13 programs, ranking 13 programs on average[9]. In comparison, the US Allopathic Seniors that went unmatched were invited to seven programs, interviewed at seven programs, and ranked all seven programs. US Osteopathic and International Graduates that matched interviewed at an average of nine programs, while those that did not match interviewed at an average of two programs.

When a program offers you an interview, after you accept the spot, you will get more specific details about the interview. Some programs will have a hotel that they use for the interview events. Other programs may be able to recommend a hotel, but do not have any specific requirements as to where you stay. You may be able to use your preferred chain of hotels where you can earn free nights. Plan on making your own travel arrangements, unless the program offers to provide assistance. If you are not familiar with the area, you can ask for advice on airports, hotels, taxis, if Uber is an option, etc.

---

[9] National Matching Residency Program (2019). *Results of the 2019 NRMP Applicant Survey by Preferred Specialty and Applicant Type*, p. 9. Retrieved from: https://mk0nrmp3oyqui6wqfm.kinstacdn.com/wp-content/uploads/2019/06/Applicant-Survey-Report-2019.pdf.

Presenting your best self

When you are preparing for your interviews, you should invest in a nice suit. A well-tailored black suit will go a long way towards setting you up for success. You can add color with your shirt and tie for men or blouse and optional scarf for women. Shoes should be black and conservative. It is advisable to look for information on dress code at the institution you are interviewing. Depending on the culture of the institution, you may wish to cover all tattoos and non-ear piercings, if the dress code requires this. Remember that while fashion for clothing and hair has changed over the decades, the professional appearance of a physician has changed very little. You can show a little personality with your hair style or color but be aware that something extreme may turn away potential programs. You can never go wrong with a traditionally professional hair style on interview day. Leave the spikes or bedhead look for another day. Keep facial hair to a minimum and well groomed.

What does it mean to be professional during your interview day and communications? It means that you present yourself in the manner a patient would expect of a physician. You should show respect for all individuals, the program, and the institution. Make sure to speak with full sentences and without slang or negative connotations. Never interrupt. Say Please and Thank You. Hold open doors for other candidates. Ask well thought-out questions. Make sure the conversation is always positive in nature. Always present yourself as a mature professional, even during breaks or social times.

The Questions

There is no way to fully prepare for the interview questions. You can be asked any number of questions. The primary interests of the programs are to learn who you are, what you know, how you learn, if you will be successful in the curriculum, and if you are a good fit for the program's culture. Interview questions tend to be open-ended and looking for either your experience or your opinion/expectations. Here are some items to think about prior to your first interview:

- Why did you choose this specialty?
- What are your expectations of what your life will be like during and after residency? Are you interested in a subspecialty?
- Are there any red flags in your application? If so, you need to have an explanation ready. Red flags include:
  - an interruption in your medical training
  - an extension of your medical training
  - a misdemeanor or felony conviction
  - failures on your medical school or USMLE/COMLEX-USA transcripts
  - previous unsuccessful training
  - previous suspended licenses
- Why should the program pick you over other candidates?
- What are your strengths?
- What is your weakness and how do you work to overcome it?
- What have you done in your life that shows that you are hardworking and dedicated?
- When have you shown informal leadership? Have you been in a position of formal leadership?
- Share a time when you demonstrated an ability to thrive under pressure.
- How do you balance personal and professional responsibilities?
- What hobbies do you have that help you to keep your work-life balance?
- If you could not be a doctor, what would you be?
- What other team-based sports or projects have you participated in? Do you prefer to work in a team or alone?
- What is the most interesting or memorable case you have seen so far?

There are hundreds of Interview questions that could be asked. You can't prepare for them all, just be yourself. Remember, this interview process is for both parties to learn more about each other. Use the time wisely to collect the information that you need to make your own decisions about the programs. Are you a good fit for the program? Do you like the city and institution? Ask all the other questions that we have discussed earlier in this book.

Ranking the Programs

After you gather all the information that you need to create your Rank List, it may be helpful to put your "rankable" programs on paper with the pros and cons to the characteristics that you prefer. I have seen some students develop a numeric system for ranking the programs. Other students have used their gut feelings about the programs they felt the most comfortable visiting and ranked those higher. You may have a certain location that you want, regardless of the program characteristics themselves. Whatever method you use, make sure that you rank ALL of the programs that you would be willing to work and train within. Do not limit yourself here.

In Tables 5-9, you can see a numeric system that I developed, which takes the guess work out of all the variables. I call it the Program Ranking Score Card Method. For each program that you are considering ranking, you complete a score card (Table 5) and compare the overall score for each program to develop a draft Rank Order List for the Match (Table 8). The program characteristics that we discussed before are summarized into categories in the score card. If you have additional categories that you would like to add, it is easy to edit this system without having to change the calculation method. This form can be used to help you create a rank order list of all the programs you are considering. I would encourage you to fill out this form for each program immediately following each interview. This will help you to analyze all the programs in a systematic way.

First, you identify the categories that are most important to you by ranking them in the first column from 1 to 12. If you would like to add other categories, you would just rank to a higher number or substitute for categories that you may not care about. This first column remains the same on every Score Card for each program that you score.

In the second column, you give each program a grade for each category using a scale of 1-3 (1: Excellent, 2: Average, 3: Below Average). Remember that a low score or placing in first place is the ideal for all of these scores.

Now that you have ranked your categories by importance and identified how the program scores in each category, you will create a special score for each program by using your importance ranking as a weight. In the third column, you multiply the Importance and Grade to fill in the Category's Score. Then, add all Category Scores to create an Overall Program Score. Table 6 and Table 7 give you examples of two program score cards filled out by a fictional medical student, Spencer. Table 9 shows the listing of all the programs that Spencer scored, which serves as a draft Rank Order List for the Match. After this list is developed, Spencer can review it and make changes based on his gut reaction. For example, he may have highly competitive programs on the top, but is he a highly competitive candidate? This method is a starting point to give you a standardized process for evaluating the programs. You can make any changes to this list based on outside influences. You can reach for the stars with a couple of competitive programs, but, if you are not a top tier candidate, make sure that you have other more reasonable choices high on your Rank Order List.

Table 5: Program Ranking Score Card (Blank)

PROGRAM RANKING SCORE CARD
PROGRAM NAME: _____

Instructions: In the first column, rank the categories by priority to you with 1-12 with 1 being the most important and 12 being the least important category of program characteristics. In the second column, grade the program on each category using a scale from 1-3 (1: Excellent, 2: Average, 3: Below Average). Multiply Important and Grade to fill in the Category Score, then add all Category Scores to create an Overall Program Score.

Importance (1-12)	Grade (1-3)	Score (I x G)	
_____	_____	_____	Accreditation status & history
_____	_____	_____	Location, cost of living, and diversity
_____	_____	_____	Quality of training and support
_____	_____	_____	Salary and benefits
_____	_____	_____	Quality of Sponsoring Institution
_____	_____	_____	Patient mix, scope, and volume
_____	_____	_____	Rotations, curriculum, call schedule, etc.
_____	_____	_____	Scholarly activity opportunities
_____	_____	_____	Current resident satisfaction
_____	_____	_____	Use of new technologies and simulations
_____	_____	_____	Program leadership
_____	_____	_____	Future opportunities after graduation

Overall Program Score =
The lower the score the better the fit of this program to your needs. Place the programs in order from lowest score to highest. This should translate to a rank list with your first program being the lowest score and your last program being the highest score.

Comments:

Table 6: Program Ranking Score Card (Sample Program A)

PROGRAM RANKING SCORE CARD
PROGRAM NAME: RESIDENCY PROGRAM A

Instructions: In the first column, rank the categories by priority to you with 1-12 with 1 being the most important and 12 being the least important category of program characteristics. In the second column, grade the program on each category using a scale from 1-3 (1: Excellent, 2: Average, 3: Below Average). Multiply Important and Grade to fill in the Category Score, then add all Category Scores to create an Overall Program Score.

Importance (1-12)	Grade (1-3)	Score (I x G)	
6	1	6	Accreditation status & history
5	1	5	Location, cost of living, and diversity
1	2	2	Quality of training and support
10	2	20	Salary and benefits
11	2	22	Quality of Sponsoring Institution
2	1	2	Patient mix, scope, and volume
3	1	3	Rotations, curriculum, call schedule, etc.
9	3	27	Scholarly activity opportunities
8	2	16	Current resident satisfaction
4	1	4	Use of new technologies and simulations
7	2	14	Program leadership
12	1	12	Future opportunities after graduation

Overall Program Score = 133

The lower the score the better the fit of this program to your needs. Place the programs in order from lowest score to highest. This should translate to a rank list with your first program being the lowest score and your last program being the highest score.

Comments:

A lot of fellowships at this institution but lacking scholarly activity. Really liked the residents and great location.

Table 7: Program Ranking Score Card (Sample Program B)

PROGRAM RANKING SCORE CARD
PROGRAM NAME: RESIDENCY PROGRAM B

Instructions: In the first column, rank the categories by priority to you with 1-12 with 1 being the most important and 12 being the least important category of program characteristics. In the second column, grade the program on each category using a scale from 1-3 (1: Excellent, 2: Average, 3: Below Average). Multiply Important and Grade to fill in the Category Score, then add all Category Scores to create an Overall Program Score.

Importance (1-12)	Grade (1-3)	Score (I x G)	
6	1	6	Accreditation status & history
5	1	5	Location, cost of living, and diversity
1	2	2	Quality of training and support
10	2	20	Salary and benefits
11	2	22	Quality of Sponsoring Institution
2	1	2	Patient mix, scope, and volume
3	1	3	Rotations, curriculum, call schedule, etc.
9	2	18	Scholarly activity opportunities
8	2	16	Current resident satisfaction
4	3	12	Use of new technologies and simulations
7	1	7	Program leadership
12	3	36	Future opportunities after graduation

Overall Program Score = 149

The lower the score the better the fit of this program to your needs. Place the programs in order from lowest score to highest. This should translate to a rank list with your first program being the lowest score and your last program being the highest score.

Comments:

No fellowships. PD is awesome. Faculty are cool. Felt very comfortable with the residents. Family like.

Table 8: Program Ranking Score Card Rank Order List (Blank)

Program Rank Order List	
Overall Program Scores	**Rank List Order** (lowest to Highest)
Program A = _____ **Program B = _____** **Program C = _____** **Program D = _____**	
Comments:	

Table 9: Program Ranking Score Card Rank Order List (Sample)

Program Rank Order List	
Overall Program Scores	**Rank List Order** (lowest to Highest)
Program A = 133 **Program B = 149** **Program C = 158** **Program D = 125** **Program E = 180** **Program F = 168** **Program G = 153** **Program H = 120** **Program I = 153**	**Program H** **Program D** **Program A** **Program B** **Program I** **Program G** **Program C** **Program F** **Program E – Do Not Rank**
Comments:	

Assuming you leave 12 categories on the Score Card, the ideal program would have an Overall Score of 78 and the worst possible program would have a score of 234. You would be advised not to consider programs that score over 175. This is not a hard cut off score, you may choose to go higher. Just be aware that below average scores are not what you want in a residency. You deserve more and should strive for more.

In this example, Spencer has interviewed in nine programs. In Table 9, you can see that the Program Ranking Score Card Method helped him determine that he wants to rank eight of these programs and not to rank one of them, because the score was 180 on that program.

Spencer has rated both Program G and Program I with 153 points. You will see that he decided to place Program I above Program G in the Rank Order List. This was because when he considered only those two programs, he felt that Program I should be ranked higher based on his overall experience with the programs.

Spencer will choose not to rank Program E, because it scored poorly across the board and he felt it was not in his best interest to attend this program.

The Match and Plan B

How it works

As you begin to develop your strategic plan for the Match process, you should review the NRMP website (www.nrmp.org). On their "How The Matching Algorithm Works" page, there is a video that provides an overview of the algorithm with a sample match. This video will be helpful for understanding the match process. The basic structure is that the applicants and the institutions all submit a Rank Order List. The process is what the NRMP calls an "applicant-proposing algorithm." Applicants are tentatively matched with the institution of their choice until another applicant is tentatively matched that is placed higher on the institution's Rank Order List. If a higher ranked applicant bumps an applicant from an institution, the next institution on their list will be reviewed for potential matching. This process continues until all applicants are run through the system and all positions are filled and/or matched completely.

There is no guarantee that all applicants will get a position. Even in the best of years, some applicants will go unmatched and some programs will go unfilled. According to the NRMP Report for Results and Data 2019, the overall PGY-1 match rate for all candidates was 79.6%.[10] For non-citizen international medical graduates, the PGY-1 match rate was 58.6%. The US Senior Allopathic School PGY-1 match rate was 93.9%. For those that graduated US Senior Allopathic Schools a year earlier or more, the match rate was only 45.4%. The US Seniors of Osteopathic School PGY-1 match rate was 84.6% for the NRMP match. This is with the Osteopathic schools still having a separate AOA match in 2019, which will not be the case in 2020.

Make sure you list as many programs as possible to increase your likelihood to match. Most importantly, be realistic with your specialty and program choices.

In 2019, there were 32,194 positions placed in the NRMP Match and 38,376 active applicants. Therefore, if all the positions filled, there would still be applicants which go unmatched. Many of these applicants are non-US citizens that graduated from international medical schools and work as physicians in their own countries. Another large group of unmatched students are US graduates who struggled to find a position directly following their senior year of medical school. In order to give yourself the best chance to match, you should rank all the programs where you would be willing to train, in the order of your preference. Make sure you list as many programs as possible to increase your

---

[10] National Matching Residency Program (2019). *Results and Data 2019 Main Residency Match*, Table 4, p. 17. Retrieved from: https://mk0nrmp3oyqui6wqfm.kinstacdn.com/wp-content/uploads/2019/04/NRMP-Results-and-Data-2019_04112019_final.pdf

likelihood to match. Most importantly be realistic with your specialty and program choices. Rank the elite program if you wish, but also rank the average programs or those in the less than ideal locations to maximize the chance that you match.

SOAP - Post Match Scramble

After the Match, there is a post-match scramble process, referred to as the Supplemental Offer and Acceptance Program (SOAP).[11] The SOAP was developed to assist applicants and programs in scrambling to fill positions which remain open after the main match process. Until a few years ago, this was a everyone fends for yourself scramble. The NRMP developed a formal process which functions like a second match, but with a different type of process which uses a rank list from the programs only. There are strict guidelines for participation in the SOAP process. All applicants must apply to programs using ERAS and are not allowed to communicate directly with the program. The programs can initiate contact with the applicants to interview or clarify application information. The institutions create a preference list for extending offers to participants. The programs can offer positions to SOAP participants in three rounds during the SOAP week. Each round is 2 hours long. The candidate can accept or reject the offer in each round. The majority of positions are filled in the first round. After SOAP week, if you are still unmatched, you may contact programs directly about unfilled positions.

What is your Plan B?

What if you can't get a residency or Transitional year position in the Match or SOAP? What options should you consider next? The first thing you should do is evaluate why you did not match. If you receive any feedback on your applications along the way, make sure you take notes.

---

[11] National Matching Residency Program (2019). *SOAP For Applicants.* Retrieved from: http://www.nrmp.org/soap-applicants-video/

Re-evaluate your specialty option. You may need to accept a different specialty in order to start a residency this year. Look for unfilled positions posted with the AMA or AOA. This is the time to swallow your pride and apply for any open positions. If you do not get a residency immediately following medical school, your chances of getting a residency in the future are significantly lower. Sometimes there are still primary care spots available after the SOAP. You would be smart to apply for one of them. With the elimination of the AOA match, we cannot predict what positions will be open after the SOAP (if any) in 2020 and beyond.

After you have exhausted all your residency options and you do not get a position, you need to implement your Plan B. Consider what you can be doing over the next year in order to improve your application for next year's match. Make sure to stay within the medical field and keep your clinical skills honed until the next match season. Depending on your state's licensing requirements, you may be able to work as a physician's assistant, Emergency Medicine Technician, or in another clinical capacity. Another option to be a research assistant in a clinical or medical setting. Use your connections to your advantage. Jump into more research projects with attending physicians. Basically, you need to keep clinically active and show your worth to potential employers during this unfortunate down time. The odds are against you for getting a residency spot after a gap year, you will need to use this year in the best possible way to maximize your next application.

One last Plan B suggestion is to make sure that you stay in connection with your favorite programs in case they have any unexpected openings in the next year. On occasion, new PGY1 residents are released from the program for any number of reasons. I have seen this happen due to difficulty in getting a license, failing a pre-employment drug or nicotine test, Visa issues, etc. If this happens, a program would rather take a previously ranked candidate over going through a whole new selection process. This is another time that your connection with the TA can be very helpful.

Ranking Tips and Tricks for a successful match
- Choose a specialty that matches your academic scores.
- Apply at multiple programs.
- Accept as many interview invitations as you can afford.
- Rank ALL reasonable programs.
  DO NOT LIMIT YOURSELF HERE!
- Rank realistic programs intermixed with "pie in the sky" programs.
- Do not accept or suggest "verbal marriages" with a program.
- Rotate to your preferred programs prior to Match season (Aug – Nov).
- Participate in the SOAP, if you go unmatched.
- Stay in touch with the program in a collegial way.
- **ALWAYS BE PROFESSIONAL!**

Chapter Six:
Coming to America
International Medical Graduates

Graduates of medical schools from outside of the USA are called International Medical graduates (IMG) or Foreign Medical Graduates (FMG). IMG is the currently preferred term used by the Educational Commission for Foreign Medical Graduates (ECFMG), but both are commonly used in GME. The ECFMG certifies IMG candidates so that they may be eligible for a US residency program. This certification includes a verification of the student's medical school training, an English language examination, and all three steps of USMLE examinations. Fundamental clinical skills are assessed using the Step 2 Clinical Skills examination. Residency programs that are ACGME accredited and supported by CMS can only accept IMGs that are ECFMG certified. Therefore, in order for an IMG to become board eligible and practice medicine in the USA, the IMG must be ECFMG certified and graduate from an ACGME accredited residency program.

Programs are not required to open positions to IMGs or foreign nationals. Some programs do not accept residency candidates that will require visa sponsorship in any way. Other programs will sponsor only specific visas. It is very important that IMGs are well versed in their visa needs so they can communicate appropriately with programs about their needs.

There are two primary visa types for foreign nationals, regardless of where they graduated medical school. The ECFMG is the official sponsor of J-1 visas. The hiring institution is the sponsor of H1-B visas.

The IMG candidate should be aware that the easiest visa option would be to have sponsorship through the ECFMG. This J-1 visa allows you to bring family members with you with their own J-2 visas. The J-1 limitation is that you are required to return to your own country for 2 years, upon residency graduation. There is a program call Conrad 30 Waiver that allows J-1 graduates to waive the 2-year residence requirements if they agree to provide medical care to patients in medically underserved areas, using a H1-B visa.[12]

A resident that plans to stay in the USA would need the sponsoring institution to sponsor an H1-B visa.[13] This is an expensive visa for the sponsor (due to legal fees) and there is significant risk to the employer if the employee does not work out (must pay to send employee home). For this reason, many institutions do not sponsor this visa or only sponsor it for hard to fill fellowships. These visas are limited in number with universities having special priority to having sponsorship approvals.

The ECFMG provides services to IMGs that will help them determine their best options and appropriate steps for acquiring a residency program. This organization should be the primary source of information for all IMGs.

Programs that are IMG friendly are often identified through the lists that you can find online. A simple google search for IMG Friendly will provide you with more than 695M links to ranking websites and resources. I would recommend that you connect with other students from your school that were successful in obtaining a US residency to find out how they identified the friendliest programs.

---

[12] U.S. Citizenship and Immigration Services (2019). *Conrad 30 Waiver Program.* Retrieved at: https://www.uscis.gov/working-united-states/students-and-exchange-visitors/conrad-30-waiver-program

[13] U.S. Citizenship and Immigration Services (2019). *Eligibility Criteria.* Retrieved at: https://www.uscis.gov/working-united-states/temporary-workers/h-1b-specialty-occupations-dod-cooperative-research-and-development-project-workers-and-fashion-models

International Medical Graduates

From the institution's standpoint, there are reasons why institutions choose to be IMG friendly and reasons why they choose not to be. The most difficult issue with hiring an IMG is that they often need visa sponsorship. In general, university-based hospitals tend to be more open to hiring IMGs in need of visa sponsorship then community hospitals. This is because universities routinely work with foreign scholars and have the expertise to process visas. Community hospitals tend to be unfamiliar with the visa sponsorship process and often lack the expertise to process these visas. Universities also have more opportunity to sponsor visas as they have difference limits on the number that the government allow them to sponsor. Even if they have the expertise, some hospitals have chosen not to sponsor H1-B visas due to the expense and risk to the hospital. The US government has enforced the requirements that the employer must pay for all fees related to the H1-B visa. This means that the employer must pay for the applicant's lawyer fees and the visa application fees. There is a requirement placed on the employer to post and verify that the employee is being paid a prevailing wage. This must be done for all locations that the employee works, which means that for every out-rotation that an IMG does during training may require additional paperwork and potentially a different wage if the rotation is in a higher wage location. In addition, the employer agrees to pay for your flight to your home country, if you do not work out as an employee. With all of the above, I believe that the expense and extra administrative work of an H1-B visa is the main reason that institutions choose not to accept IMGs.

Some institutions will accept IMGs with J-1 visas . This visa is sponsored by the ECFMG and only requires a single form to be filed upon arrival of the resident and when they leave. However, many institutions are seriously hoping to retain their residents upon graduation and this type of visa generally does not allow for the resident to remain with the institution as an attending physician.

Candidates should know that institutions that support IMGs often do so because they appreciate the expertise and quality that IMGs can bring to their programs. Many IMGs are fully licensed practicing physicians in their own countries. It is reasonable to say that due to sheer experience, IMGs can come to the US and function at a much higher level than a recent US graduate.

There are a several areas that institutions have historically had issues with IMGs. It is important that I mention them here, so you can determine if you need to make improvements prior to interviewing: Communication and Cultural integration. IMGs often learn English as a secondary language. This can lead to strong accents and difficulty in understanding between peers from different countries. In addition, patients can have difficulty understanding the resident, especially older patients with poor hearing and limited experience with accents. A quality IMG who wishes to maximize their communication will:

- Work diligently to minimize strong accents
- Speak clearly and succinctly
- Learn local slang to better communicate with patients
- Be well versed in English medical terminology

The US culture is very different from other countries and can be very different from one state to another. However, two cultural competency issues that we see with IMGs across the country are equality and sexual harassment. These are often connected issues. When an IMG comes from a country where one sex has authority over the other sex, the individual may have difficulty with treating all individuals equally. In truth, they often do not realize that they are treating people unequally until it is pointed out to them. If they are not careful, the IMG may be labeled as chauvinist or an elitist. An IMG can often get into trouble for making comments related to the opposite sex, without realizing that those comments rise to the level of sexual harassment. Institutions provide sexual harassment training to all employees to ensure that all employees understand definitions and expectations to minimize issues in this area. A successful resident will be aware of these concerns and work diligently to ensure that he/she is never placed in a position of being accused of such behavior.

Chapter Seven:
I Matched, Now What?
The Onboarding Process

Once you match with a program, you will receive a welcome email congratulating you on matching to their program. Each institution and program have their own onboarding process. Some programs use online technology, giving you access to an online database where you will upload your documents and complete assignments. Other programs will ask you to complete documents and return them to the training administrator.

Check your email daily for new information from the program. The program has ten (10) days in which to send you a contract for your signature. You need to review it for accurate name, specialty program, salary, dates, etc. This contract is not negotiable, so you only have the option of clarifying your personal information. If you have any questions about the contract, you should ask the person that sent it to you. It should not be significantly different from the sample contract that you received while interviewing with the program. However, it is common for the salary to increase or for small changes to occur between recruitment season and contract signing.

The contract will probably have a July 1 start date and be for a full year. You should be asked to sign another contract every year of your training. If there are any changes to your contracted dates, a simple contract addendum is likely to be created for your signature. However, I have seen hospitals that change dates using a formal letter from the PD to the resident. If you are required to attend an orientation prior to beginning your residency, the contract may include one or two weeks in the end of June prior to your program start date. The orientation dates do not need to be included on your residency program contract, but you will be required to attend. Make sure that you pay close attention to the details on when you must report for orientation.

Expect to do some work prior to arriving at your residency. You will be required to complete the training for Basic Life Support (BLS) and Advanced Cardiac Life Support (ACLS) certification. Your medical school or your residency program may provide you with this training. In some cases, you will be expected to arrive with the certification on your own. You may also need to complete applications for educational licensure, get your fingerprints taken for background checks, obtain your National Provider Identification (NPI) number, complete program and institutional specific documents, provide certificates and diplomas, and often complete online compliance training prior to arriving onsite.

Expect to do some work prior to arriving at your residency.

It may seem strange, but some institutions will have a Human Resources (HR) representative contact you to "offer you the job." This is a formality after the Match, since the Match is a binding commitment that only the NRMP can break as long as you are compliant with all institutional policies for new hires. When HR contacts you, there is usually a time clock that starts for you to have a drug test done for hiring purposes. They will provide you with instructions to have this drug testing and may require you to come into Employee Health for a simple "fit for duty" physical. When you live a significant distance from the institution which you will be joining, you will do the drug test locally right away and can often arrange for the physical during or just before orientation week when you have moved into town.

The Onboarding Process

It is very important to understand the HR policies that relate to your hiring into the institution. Matching does not protect you from losing the position, if you do not meet their hiring criteria or the state's licensing requirements. I have personally seen new residents lose their positions because of positive drug tests, positive nicotine tests, and inability to obtain a medical license. Recently, some states have legalized marijuana. Smoking and drinking alcohol are also legal activities. Some employers have strict policies about these substances. Having these "legal" substances in your blood can be a cause for denying you a residency position, regardless of the Match results.

Matching does not protect you from losing the position, if you do not meet their hiring criteria or the state's licensing requirements.

When you are ready to look for housing, the program or institution may offer some assistance. They can recommend safe and reasonably priced neighborhoods. They may have connections with realtors. They also may have listings posted within their department of houses for sale by graduating residents. When you pick a place to live, you will need to provide proof of employment. The training administrator can provide you with a letter of employment that can be used to apply for a mortgage or rent approval. You can use your contract, but it is easier and more private to provide a single page letter for this purpose. Plan to move into town at least one or two weeks before you begin orientation. You will want to be settled into your new place before you start, because you will have very little time to settle in after you begin. It is best to look for housing which would be available in early to mid-June and within a reasonably short commute to the hospital.

As you become an upperclassman, you may have the opportunity to take call from home. If your program offers this option, you will be required to live within a specific time distance from the hospital. Most institutions mandate that someone on home call can arrive within 20-30 minutes. Take this into consideration when you decide on your new residence. I have seen married residents, that are in programs more than an hour apart from each other, choose to live right in the middle. This meant that they both had a 45-minute commute and were not eligible for home call in their senior years. If this happens, you would have to take call within the hospital or stay somewhere closer to the hospital on your call nights. You can safely assume that your work hours will be long and that you will, on occasion, be tired while driving to and from work. Add the factor that you will sometimes have bad weather and it is reasonable to say that it is safer for you and those around you, if you have a short commute, specifically if you need to drive your own car.

One last recommendation on finding a place to live is to ask around for information on the areas to consider. The current residents, faculty, and staff can tell you where the best areas are close to the hospital or university. They can also advise you on the areas to avoid for safety and/or resale reasons. I had one resident that lived in a rather unsafe area, because he did not even consider this factor. He just looked at price and apartment size. He was stuck in a lease for a full year and somewhat uncomfortable coming and going at the odd hours that his training required. Sometimes, graduating residents will be looking for someone to purchase their house, so it does not hurt to touch base with the residents and ask. You may find an ideal house close by with no real estate commissions to pay.

Orientation

You will be provided with a date, time, and location to appear for orientation. A full itinerary may not be shared until you arrive. You can expect orientation to be exciting and boring at the same time. You are excited to get to know your peers and get started as a resident.

However, you must go through a process of learning a bunch of important but boring stuff. So, what can you expect?

Arrive at least 10-15 minutes early, especially if you have never been to this room before. Dress professionally (like you would for clinic) unless you are told otherwise. Some institutions will allow business casual or casual dress on certain days. Bring a pen. You will be provided with schedules, logins, maybe final forms to fill out, etc. Make sure that you have a way of taking notes and as you go through the sessions, write down any questions that you have. Orientation is often broken down into institutional and program sessions. At the institutional orientation sessions, you will be with all PGY1 residents entering the institution. You will probably meet representatives from multiple areas of the hospital, such as human resources, risk/compliance, physician leaders, administration, pharmacy, graduate medical education, nursing, etc. These are often simple meet and greet sessions. Sometimes these include a 30-60 minutes presentation with highlights on what you need to know. These can get tedious and, yes, I will admit boring. Over the years, most institutions have limited these sessions to the bear minimum of "must haves" for new residents. Some "must haves" are dictated by accreditation requirements, so even though you don't feel it was necessary...it was.

Do yourself a favor - put the phone away and silence it

Remember that this is the first time you are in front of some of these leaders. You want to be respectful during all these orientation sessions. Even if you are not asked to do so, turn off your phone or put it on complete silent mode. Even a vibrating phone can interrupt the speaker. Some speakers will see a resident on his phone and believe that he is not listening. I have seen residents get bad reputations on day one because of this. We have even had formal conversations with residents about putting their phone away and paying attention to the speaker. If you plan to take notes on your phone, you should ask your TA prior to orientation if this would be acceptable. By asking, you are making it known that you are not texting or playing games but taking notes during the orientation session. This is the only reason that a phone should be in sight of the speaker. If you are not using it to take notes, you should have it away, so that it does not distract you with non-orientation business.

Often orientation week is a time to get to know your peers and fellow residents at social events. It is common to have at least one formal social event. This can be attending a local professional baseball game, backyard barbeques with your program director and faculty, formal or informal welcome receptions, or team building events such as an escape room, golf, or a bowling competition. You should make sure that you participate in these events, even if they are optional. It is a place to make connections that will be very beneficial for your residency. Social events often are the only opportunity for spouses and significant others to meet the team, so include them when they are invited as well.

Make sure that you get answers to all your questions during orientation. It is very important that you understand what expectations are placed on you for the next year. Here are a few questions that you should be able to answer after orientation.

- Who do I call if I am sick and unable to come into work?
- Do I need to contact a senior resident prior to the start of a new rotation?
- What is my daily schedule for rotation #1?
- Where do I report on July 1? What time?
- Am I on-call this month? What is expected of me while on-call? Do I report to a specific person at a specific time in a specific location for call shifts?
- How do I log my work hours and procedure logs?

- What reading should I be doing and when?
- What events must I attend outside of my assigned rotation? (i.e. Journal Club, program specific didactic sessions, Grand Rounds, hospital wide events)
- If my rotation activities conflict with my program activities, which takes precedence? If you will miss the program's events for a rotation event (or vice versa), make sure that you inform the appropriate person of the conflict and necessary absence.
- Was my license issued, so I can start on July 1?
- Do I owe any paperwork or proof of training to HR or GME?
- Do I need to register for any federal or state databases to treat patients? For example, in order to treat Medicare patients, you need to be registered in the Medicare Provider and Supplier (PECOS) database through the Centers for Medicare and Medicaid Services.

Take III

Now that you are either waiting to start or just started your residency, it is time to take your USMLE III or COMLEX-USA III examination. It is best to take this examination earlier, rather than later. You will be sleep deprived and very busy in your PGY1 year. If you have a month or two off before you start residency, you could use this time to study and take this examination. The score is not as big of an issue as for the I and II examinations. The score needs to be a passing score for licensure reasons. However, unless you are looking for a fellowship, the actual numerical score will be irrelevant, as long as it is a passing score.

Many students take a long vacation right after medical school graduation. If you are burnt out from medical school, give yourself a break. As soon as you can take the examination after your break, do it. If you wait until you are in your PGY1 or PGY2 years, be strategic and plan to take the examination during a rotation where you can take several days off at a time. I suggest it during an emergency medicine rotation, since this rotation is often set up in shifts and you can rearrange your shifts to have several days off for the examination. Ask your TA if you have paid administrative leave for this examination or if you have to take vacation time.

You will have until the end of your PGY2 year to successfully complete the third examination. If you are not successful in USMLE III or COMLEX-USA III, you cannot move into your third year. By taken the examination early, you will allow yourself plenty of time to retake the examination if you have difficulty with passing. When you pass the examination, you must provide proof to your residency program, so it can be added to your academic record. You should be able to provide this evidence by March of your PGY2 year, so that you can receive your PGY3 contract in the spring with your peers.

Chapter Eight:
Residency Basics

Clinical and Education Work Hours

You will need to log your hours throughout your training. You will be oriented on the requirements as you enter your program. Basically, you cannot work more than 80 hours per week averaged over a four-week period, with some exceptions. This includes all in-house clinical and educational activities, time spent on clinical work when at home, and all moonlighting hours. You cannot moonlight during your first year of training. Moonlighting as a PGY2 or higher is dependent upon approval by your PD. Some programs do not allow moonlighting, so you will concentrate on your program only.

The reason for these duty hour restrictions is to ensure that residents are not forced to work too many hours, causing you to be fatigued during patient care, studying, or during transportation. In addition, you will receive training on fatigue mitigation and sleep hygiene (tips for getting better sleep).

There are additional rules that mandate a minimum of one day off in every seven days (averaged over a four-week period), maximum lengths of shifts, limitations on night float shifts, and call shifts. You will be instructed on how to log your hours and what specific rules your program has related to those logs. Please make sure that you are accurate in your logging. If you have a policy violation once, it is not a big issue. However, if it is a pattern, the log should indicate this. The PD or TA will be reviewing your work hour logs routinely. If they see a pattern, they can address it. If they do not have the information, they cannot address it.

When multiple residents are having extended hours in the same rotation, this gives the PD the necessary documentation to address the issue. In this case, the PD should speak with the rotation preceptors to determine if a schedule change is needed. If the PD is not provided the correct information in the log, the PD is not able to address issues of non-compliance by the rotation schedules. Do not assume that your PD knows about the issues, make sure that the documentation shows clearly what hours violations need to be addressed.

Rotation schedules

When you attend orientation, you will be provided with an annual rotation schedule. You should review this schedule to ensure that it meets all your educational needs. I suggest that you review the schedule along with the ACGME's curriculum requirements for your specialty. Your TA and program director would have created this schedule with your required rotations in mind, but errors do occur. After you verify that you have the correct rotations scheduled, you will want to determine if you have any special events happening where you will need time off work. If you have a sibling getting married and must have 3 days off to participate, make sure that you bring this information to the TA and PD right away. You may be told that specific rotations do not allow vacation, or you may be assigned to a night shift when you need an evening off. These situations can be addressed most efficiently when you bring them forward at the beginning of the year. TAs will work with you to address your vacation needs, sometimes switching rotations in order to do so.

Review your rotation schedule and ask for time off to attend special events at the beginning of the year when you can.

During your program, you will have several opportunities to choose elective rotations. Some PGY1 years will allow elective rotations, but often electives are in the later years. Ask your TA if there are any policies that relate to your elective choices. Some programs will offer a specific set of options, while others will consider options brought forward by the resident. Most institutions will limit your electives to being within the hospital and its affiliated clinics. On occasion, an elective out-rotation will be considered for educational reasons, such as rural medicine or a subspecialty experience in your field. Your TA can give you examples of the electives that have been approved in the past.

So, what is identified as an out-rotation and why is this important to the resident? In general, a rotation is considered an out-rotation when it takes place in another teaching hospital or at a clinical site that is not directly affiliated with your sponsoring institution. There are two types of out-rotations: required and elective. Required rotations are part of the standard curriculum where all residents attend the rotation during the training program. An elective rotation is a rotation that a single or several residents may attend, but not required by the program.

For required out-rotations, a resident goes to another clinical site that is not under the administrative oversight of the sponsoring institution or primary teaching site and a formal relationship is identified between the hosting institution and the program. This formal relationship is documented in a Program Letter of Agreement (PLA), which identifies the goals and objectives for the rotation. Different specialties have different expectations on when a PLA is necessary. The PLA must be an agreement between your PD and the outside training site faculty supervisor. The Sponsoring Institution's DIO is often a signatory on this agreement as well. PLAs are considered optional for electives in many specialties. However, regardless of whether a PLA is necessary, most sponsoring institutions will require an affiliation agreement with malpractice insurance and corporate risk clauses. For this reason, the TA needs to be aware of potential elective rotations at least three to six months in advance, so the proper procedure for authorization and approval can begin. When you are assigned to attend an out-rotation, regardless of whether it is elective or required, you will need to consider a few items.

- Is it within driving distance of your home? If it is more than one hour away, you should stay at a closer location. If this is a required rotation, your program may have funds identified to assist with these expenses.
- Is it in the same state? If not, you will need to apply for a temporary educational license in the state of the rotation.
- Who is submitting the paperwork to the host institution? Are you the primary contact for scheduling and applying for the rotation or is your TA going to handle this? There is usually a list of documents that the institution will require prior to your arrival. They may also require you to do additional training for the rotation prior to arrival. For example, if it is a trauma surgery rotation, you may need to take Advanced Trauma Life Support (ATLS) prior to arrival.
- If you are requesting an elective, you may be required to submit a statement of educational merit to receive authorization from the PD and GME office.

Certifications and Licenses

The TA will be your partner in making sure that you have all your documentation up-to-date and that you remain compliant with all policies and procedures. Always look at communications from your TA. Most TAs provide reminders of requirement and deadlines, because they understand that residents have a lot on their minds. You will begin residency with BLS and ACLS certification which will need to be renewed every two years. You have state and possibly federal licenses (medical and pharmaceutical) that will need annual updates while in the educational stage. The TA can help you determine when you qualify for a more permanent license and can assist you in applying for your licenses. In addition, you may have specialty specific licenses or certifications that your TA will track for you. Make sure that you communicate routinely with your TA about any requirements and what you need to do to remain compliant. While the TA will gladly assist you, YOU are ultimately responsible for making sure you complete all necessary documentation and training, so make sure you are well aware of the requirements and verify that everything has been received and documented appropriately.

Open Enrollment

For many of you, this will be your first full-time job with benefits. One very important annual event that you need to understand is *Open Enrollment*. Each year, you can make changes to your employee benefits such as insurance (health, dental, and vision), medical savings plans, life insurance, and/or investment plans. There are two ways that Open Enrollment happens, active or passive. In active enrollments, you must re-enlist for the benefits in order to keep them. In passive enrollments, you only need to do something if you want to change something. Your employer may have either version of Open Enrollment or a combination of both.

Pay attention to Open Enrollment deadlines &
ALWAYS report qualifying life events
within 30 days to update insurance

It may seem strange that you sign up for benefits when you begin in July, then are asked to sign up again within six months. Remember that you must sign up annually for benefits and this sign up is based on the fiscal year of the employer, not your hire date. Therefore, the re-enrollment is likely to be in the middle of your first academic year. Make sure that you do not miss these deadlines. Another important deadline that you need to be aware of is that you only have thirty (30) days to make changes to your health insurance based on major events in your life, otherwise known as 'qualifying events'. These qualifying events include changes in marital status and the birth or adoption of a child.

Unfortunately, when you get busy in your residency, it is easy to forget to update your benefits through HR. This has happened too many times in my career. Let me share three stories with you.

Case #1 - Dr. Scott

Dr. Scott is expecting his first child with his wife. He does not mention anything to his TA about the pending birth. The baby is born pre-mature at another hospital and Dr. Scott takes a week of vacation to spend some time in the neonatal unit (NICU) with the baby. He does not share the reason for his quick vacation request, other than a family emergency. The baby spends five weeks in the hospital. Dr. Scott is worried that if he asks for more time off, he will not be supported by his PD or fellow residents as he is in a very competitive residency. Scott returns to work after his week of vacation, spending every minute that he can with his wife and newborn at the hospital across town after working all day. Once the baby is released to home, Dr. Scott shares with his TA that this was all a terrifying situation and he is glad he got through it successfully. The TA asks if he contacted HR to add the baby to his health insurance. He had not even considered that. He was too tired and worried to think about such a thing. He asked if he can get an exemption from the 30-day deadline, due to his special circumstances. The TA informed the DIO, who called the VP of Human Resources. The answer was that the deadline is mandated by the federal government. The employer does not have any opportunity to grant special exemptions. Dr. Scott was responsible for the entire bill for the baby's care while in the hospital. In addition, because open enrollment was another five months away, there was no financial coverage for months of well-baby visits and immunizations. In this case, Dr. Scott's institutional leaders were able to work with the NICU hospital to arrange for a discount in the fees, but Dr. Scott still had a significant debt due to missing the insurance deadline. If While Dr. Scott was aware of this policy from orientation, it never occurred to him to mention the baby to the TA. If he had, the TA may have been able to remind him of the deadline and go over how he needed to report the birth.

Case #2 – Dr. Justin

Dr. Justin was expecting his second child with his wife, while in his third year of residency. He informed the PD and TA that he would like to have paternal leave upon the arrival of the baby. The PD placed Justin on a rotation where he could be pulled from the rotation without issue at a moment's notice with backup plans for coverage. The vacation was approved with the dates open ended. The TA provided Dr. Justin with a reminder that he needed to notify HR within 30 days of the birth. Once the baby is born, Dr. Justin takes a two-week vacation. Upon his return, the TA asks if he contacted HR yet. He states that he forgot. The TA provides him with the form to fill in the new beneficiary information. Dr. Justin fills in the form and faxes it to HR right away. All expense of the baby's birth and well-baby medical care was covered by insurance.

Case #3 – Dr. Cassie

Dr. Cassie is a resident that finds out that she is expecting. She waits until the second trimester to tell anyone, then she comes into the TA's office to let her know she will need to take the rest of her vacation when the baby is born. The TA gives Dr. Cassie a copy of the employer's policy for the Family Medical Leave Act (FMLA). Dr. Cassie states, "I will only take the vacation that I have outstanding, so I will not need to sign up for

FMLA." The TA informs her that FMLA is not optional, it is a requirement by federal law, and it is meant to protect her in case she needs more time off. In addition, this employer offers short term disability insurance. So, in Dr. Cassie's case, if she completes the FMLA paperwork and the STD paperwork, she can take up to six weeks off. Three weeks would be vacation with full pay and weeks four through six would be with partial paychecks (40% for this policy). Dr. Cassie decides to take advantage of this option and signs up for both FMLA and STD. If Dr. Cassie would have needed more time due to a medical issue, she could have received it using unpaid leave under the FMLA, up to 12 weeks in total. When Dr. Cassie has the baby, the TA reaches out via email to remind her to contact HR to enroll the baby on insurance. Dr. Cassie completes the enrollment from home via a phone call to HR and follow-up documentation. When Dr. Cassie returned to her residency rotations, she sat down with the TA to determine how many days needed to be made up to cover the additional time off, above and beyond her vacation time. As she took three additional weeks off, the PD and TA calculated that her advancement date needed to be pushed back three weeks. Her rotation and call schedule were rearranged to accommodate the new date. All expenses of the baby's birth and well-baby medical care was covered by insurance.

I share these stories to provide you with an example of why it is beneficial to share some personal information with your TA and PD. These individuals can really look out for you and make sure that you address any issues before they become problems. Anytime that you think your schedule may change or you have a major life change, you should have a conversation with either your TA or PD as a heads up. They can often fix problems before they happen, but only if they are aware of the issues.

Supervision

While you are a resident, you should never be left alone for patient care. You should always have some sort of supervision. You should always have someone to call on, if you need assistance or are unsure what to do next. The ACGME identifies four levels of supervision in the Common Program Requirements for Residency (VI.A.2.c.).[14] The levels of supervision identify the role of a supervising physician. This supervising physician may be a faculty member, an authorized senior resident, or a fellow. The level of supervision and the identified supervisor will be based on the needs of the patient and the skills of the individual resident. The progressive levels of supervision are:

- Direct Supervision - a supervising physician is physically present with the resident and patient.
- Indirect On-Site Supervision - indirect Supervision, with a supervising physician physically within the hospital or patient care site and immediately available.
- Indirect Off-Site Supervision - indirect Supervision, with a supervising physician available via phone or electronic means, but not physically present.
- Oversight Supervision – After patient care is delivered, the supervising physician reviews the encounter with feedback.

You will begin your residency with Direct supervision and progressively move through Indirect On-Site, Indirect Off-Site, and then to Oversight Supervision. Notice that there is no level called "independent" in the Common Program Requirements. All patient care remains at the "Oversight" level after the resident proves competent in providing the

---

[14] ACGME Common Program Requirements (Residency), July 2019, p.37-38. Found at: https://acgme.org/Portals/0/PFAssets/ProgramRequirements/CPRResidency2019.pdf

care or treatment. While you are a trainee, all care that you provide is under the supervision of a fully licensed attending physician. Even if you are supervised by a senior resident, they are still supervised by a licensed attending physician. The attending (faculty) physician is ultimately responsible for the patient care that is provided under their supervision.

Your institution should have a process to track your training progress and determine your required level of supervision for common procedures that you may perform. Make sure that you know this process and that you follow the necessary steps to advance to the next level of supervision in a timely manner. Your advancement in this area will be tracked by your program director and may affect your promotion date.

Be very careful to stay inside the scope of practice lines of your rotation for your own legal protection.

One last important tip regarding supervision is to make sure your supervisor is privileged in the area that they are supervising. You will learn more about scope of practice and privileging in our next book. Basically, a physician is given permission to provide very specific medical care to patients in a hospital, referred to as "scope of practice." While working with faculty members, you cannot do something under their supervision that is not in their scope of practice. You may have the experience and knowledge to do the procedure or task, but if you are not assigned to that rotation with those faculty supervising you, you may not be able to do that procedure, unless it is an emergency situation. For example, you cannot do a surgical procedure while on a non-surgical rotation. It is helpful to remember what rotation you are on and what your rotation's faculty do within their scope of practice. If you need to go outside the scope of your current rotation for emergency purposes, make sure that you are credentialed to complete the necessary task and follow up immediately with a properly privileged supervisor for that task or procedure.

Also, remember that private practice and hospital practice are different. A private physician that works within the hospital may have different scope of practice limitations in the hospital than in the private clinic. It is always safer to ask your faculty member before you move into a questionable area of practice. Hopefully, the faculty member will know his or her responsibilities for scope of practice and can guide you in what you can and cannot do under their supervision. Do not put yourself at risk. While I am not a lawyer, I have been told by lawyers that performing a procedure on a patient where you are not properly supervised by a privileged attending can place you in legal jeopardy. In addition, if you practice medicine while you are unlicensed, you can be legally accused of assault. Therefore, you cannot start your residency clinical training until your license is active. Be very careful to stay inside the scope of practice lines for your own protection. If you ever have any questions about this or other legal gray areas, consult your Compliance and Risk Officer. They are there to protect you legally.

Assessment and Evaluations

While you are in residency, you will have structured reading and unstructured reading. You will have didactic (classroom learning) sessions where you will discuss the formal curriculum items with your peers and faculty. You will have designated sessions for review of journals and scholarly activity. In addition, you will be expected to read for your current rotation as well. If you are on a general surgery, you should be reading about the cases you will be participating in during the next day's operations.

You will be tested annually with an in-service or in-training examination. This is an examination that is given annually to all residents. It is specialty specific and training level specific. The program director or program staff will moderate a standardized testing environment where you will be given a set time period to complete the examination. You should receive information regarding your raw score and your percentile score compared to all residents in your training year for that specialty. The program director is looking for a high percentile and an overall increase from year to year. Programs cannot use a low score as the <u>only</u> reason for not promoting you to the next level of training. However, a low score can be an indication that you are not learning the curriculum and need further assistance. Together with other evaluations, this can lead to academic remediation or probation. The overall performance of the program's residents on the in-training examinations provides the program with an assessment of program educational quality. Therefore, it is very important to study for these tests and attempt to do your best for every one of these assessments.

In residency, you will be evaluated differently than you were in your student years. You will receive Goals and Objectives for each of your rotations. At the end of your rotation, your faculty will evaluate your performance based on the goals and objectives of the rotation. This is commonly referred to as the monthly evaluation. You will meet with your program director or a faculty mentor every 3-6 months to review your performance. This will include a review of your procedure logs, case logs, exam scores, simulation assessments, and general performance.

ACGME Core Competencies

The ACGME had specific outcomes-based milestones categorized within six core competencies that you will need to meet during your residency training. These milestones are reported to the ACGME every six (6) months. First, let's identify the core competency categories, then we will discuss milestones. These Competencies are a conceptual framework to identify the necessary skills and knowledge for an autonomous physician across all specialties. These Core Competencies were developed and implemented in 1999[15]. Specific details can be reviewed in Section IV.B of the ACGME Common Program Requirements[16].

Below are very brief descriptors of the six ACGME Core Competency categories:
- Patient Care and Procedural Skills
  o Effectively treating patients with compassion and appropriate care
  o Ability to perform all procedures for specialty
- Medical Knowledge
  o Demonstrate evolving knowledge for specialty
  o Appropriate application of medical knowledge
- Practice-based Learning and Improvement
  o Using your knowledge, investigating, and evaluating new information to care for your patients.
  o Using new research and continuously improvement in the care of patients
  o Lifelong learning and self-evaluation
- Interpersonal and Communication Skills
  o Effective exchange of information with all stakeholders
  o Educating patients
  o Consulting with and for other caregivers

---

[15] Laura Edgar, Sydney Roberts, and Eric Holmboe (2018) Milestones 2.0: A Step Forward. Journal of Graduate Medical Education: June 2018, Vol. 10, No. 3, pp. 367-369. https://doi.org/10.4300/JGME-D-18-00372.1
[16] ACGME Common Program Requirements (Residency), July 2019, p.18-22. Found at: https://acgme.org/Portals/0/PFAssets/ProgramRequirements/CPRResidency2019.pdf

- o Maintaining comprehensive, accurate, and complete medical records
- o Working with patients and family to assess care goals
- Professionalism
    - o Commitment to professionalism
    - o Ethical principles and practices
    - o Responsiveness to patients that supersedes self-interest
    - o Respect for patient and accountability to patient, society, and the profession
    - o Personal well-being
    - o Cultural competency and responsiveness
    - o Integrity and compassion
- Systems-based Practice
    - o Ability to use the resources of the healthcare system for optimal health care of your patient
    - o Coordination of resources with an understanding of what you can and cannot do for your patient
    - o Working well within the healthcare team
    - o Understanding financial impacts on patient decisions
    - o Advocating for your patients within the system

ACGME Milestones

In 2013, with the implementation of what was called the Next Accreditation System, Milestones were added to the competencies to give specific goals, within each of the competencies, that were specialty specific. The ACGME has developed a *Milestones Guidebook for Residents and Fellows* that is available on the resident portion of their website. This guide goes through the philosophy of the milestones and how they are used. The original milestones are being revised. By the end of 2020, all specialties are supposed to be functioning with the second generation of milestones, referred to as "Milestones 2.0"[17]. So, what are milestones and how will you be evaluated for them?

In order to answer this question, it is simplest to explain milestones with child development. Think back to your pediatrics rotation. When you are evaluating a baby's development, you review specific measurable goals, such as height and weight. From this data, you determine the child's percentile in height and weight. This information tells you if the child is lacking essentials for proper brain and body development. You also look for new skills (crawling, standing, walking, etc.) and new communication and behavioral skills (talking, understanding behavior expectations, etc.) to determine if the child is developing on track.

The basics for child development assessment and the measurement of milestones in residency are similar concepts. In residency, you are assessed for measurable goals with the in-training examination, where your percentile score is compared to others in your training level. You are expected to achieve certain behavioral and skill-based milestones as you progress through your training. Do you see the correlation?

Having milestones identified for each specialty helps each program within that specialty to be addressing the same goals. It helps the faculty to understand what they need to teach and the residents to understand what they need to learn. The milestones also lay out a general expectation of the steps towards the final goal. For example, returning to our child development example, you would not expect a baby to ride a bike. In childhood, you must crawl before riding a bike, so crawling and walking would be lower scores on the physical milestone, where you may be striving years later to ride the bike with training wheels first and then independently.

---

17 Laura Edgar, Sydney Roberts, and Eric Holmboe (2018) Milestones 2.0: A Step Forward. Journal of Graduate Medical Education: June 2018, Vol. 10, No. 3, pp. 367-369. https://doi.org/10.4300/JGME-D-18-00372.1

Below is an example of a General Surgery milestone from version 2.0.[18] This example is provided for the sole purpose of educating you on what a milestone looks like and how it is scored by your faculty. You can see this specific milestone is in the Professionalism Competency. The Milestone is for Professional Behavior and Accountability.

Table 10: General Surgery Milestone Sample

Professionalism 2: Professional Behavior and Accountability				
Level 1	Level 2	Level 3	Level 4	Level 5
Completes patient care tasks and responsibilities, identifies potential barriers, and describes strategies for ensuring timely task completion	Performs patient care tasks and responsibilities in a timely manner with appropriate attention to detail in routine situations	Performs patient care tasks and responsibilities in a timely manner with appropriate attention to detail in complex or stressful situations	Recognizes situations that may impact others' ability to complete patient-care tasks and responsibilities in a timely manner	Develops systems to enhance other's ability to efficiently complete patient-care tasks and responsibilities
Describes when and how to appropriately report lapses in professional behavior	Takes responsibility for his or her own professional behavior	Demonstrates professional behavior in complex or stressful situations	Intervenes to prevent and correct lapses in professional behavior in self and others Appropriately reports lapses in professional behavior (simulated or actual)	Coaches others when their behavior fails to meet professional expectations
Recognizes limits in the knowledge/skills of self and seeks help	Recognizes limits in the knowledge/skills of team and seeks help	Exhibits appropriate confidence and self-awareness of limits in knowledge/skills	Aids junior learners in recognition of limits in knowledge/skills	

Comments:

Not Yet Completed Level 1 ☐

There are five levels identified, but there are ten potential scores. You can either score below 1, at 1, between 1 and 2, at 2, between 2 and 3, and so on. Scoring at the level means that you meet every expectation listed within that level. If you meet some items in the next level, but not all items, you score between the levels. In general, you should reach the 4th level of each milestone by graduation in order to successfully practice

---

[18] ACGME, Surgery Milestones 2.0 (January 2019), page 13. Found at: https://acgme.org/Portals/0/PDFs/Milestones/SurgeryMilestones2.0.pdf?ver=2019-05-29-124604-347

medicine independently. You may even reach the 5th level for some milestones. However, there is no requirement to get to level 4 by graduation. Your program director determines if you have met his/her expectations for graduation independent of this score. This is a tool used by the program to gauge your advancement through the milestones. However, your scores are reported to the ACGME every six months.

Clinical Competency Committee

Your program director is responsible for determining your level of promotion and when you will promote to the next training level in the program or to graduation. However, he does not work in a bubble. He has a group of faculty members that help advise him on each trainee's performance. This group is called the Clinical Competency Committee (CCC). The CCC has core faculty members, of which both physician and non-physician faculty can participate. The TA documents all meetings. The Chairperson should not be the PD, it should be a core faculty member that is well versed in ACGME assessment methods and expectations. The CCC meets at least every six months to review all resident performance and to score the residents' milestones. The PD should attend this meeting, so he hears all the information shared about resident performance.

Reporting Structure

While the PD is responsible for determining your progression in the program, with the advisement of the CCC, he/she is not completely autonomous. If the PD decides to place someone on remediation or probation, this is a reportable event to the Graduate Medical Education Committee or at least to the DIO. The DIO is the individual with the authority and responsibility for overseeing the Sponsoring Institution's ACGME accredited programs. Above the DIO, the Sponsoring

Institution's governing body (i.e. board of directors) has the 'ultimate authority' over GME at the institution. This multiple layer reporting structure protects the residents from a rogue program director or faculty member holding back promotions or forcing a probation without merit. If you ever have issues within the program, always bring the issues to your PD's attention, then to the DIO. In addition, the Graduate Medical Education Committee (GMEC) and the Sponsoring Institution's governing board would be able to address issues, after you have exhausted your options with the PD and DIO. If after all those options, you still feel you need resolution, you can call the ACGME, either anonymously or as a whistleblower. Never go to the ACGME without exhausting all opportunities for resolution at the sponsoring institution. Involving the ACGME could bring red flags to light and may negatively affect your program's accreditation.

Resident/Fellow Forum

The ACGME Institutional Requirements (II.C) has a specific clause that requires each sponsoring institution to provide an opportunity for trainees across all programs to come together without administrators.[19] The event is called a Resident/Fellow Forum. At the Forum, any resident or fellow can raise concerns to other residents/fellows in attendance. These concerns are summarized by resident representatives and presented to the DIO and GMEC. Some concerns are shared for informational purposes only, while others are issues that need to be addressed. Many institutions have created a student government or Resident/Fellow Council to run these forums. Often the resident representatives on the Council are the same that sit on the GMEC. All accredited programs should be invited to participate in the Council and

---

[19] ACGME Institutional Requirements (2018), p. 6. Found at: https://acgme.org/Portals/0/PFAssets/InstitutionalRequirements/000InstitutionalRequirements2018.pdf?ver=2018-02-19-132236-600

Forum. If you would like to get involved in leadership, this is a great opportunity.

Site Visits

The ACGME provides accreditation oversight via a specialty specific oversight committee called the Review Committee (RC). Each specialty has its own RC that reviews the data submitted to the ACGME and makes determinations on accreditation status. In addition, there is an Institutional RC that has oversight over sponsoring institution accreditation. Another separately run committee collects and analyzes data on the Clinical Learning Environment (CLE) of all GME sponsoring institutions. The CLE committee does not have accreditation oversight but is advising the ACGME on improvements that are needed for the national clinical learning environment.

These two committees, the RC and the CLE, each have their own type of inspections, called site visits. You are very likely to participate in at least one during your tenure. The first type of visit is a site visit regarding the accreditation of the program or sponsoring institution. This happens more frequently in new programs or institutions and then moves to a ten-year cycle for established programs. However, when there are concerns that arise in information that is routinely submitted to the Review Committee (RC), an impromptu site visit can be scheduled. A site visit may arise from resident concerns or complaints as well.

A Site visit from the RC involves the TA pulling together a large amount of documentation from resident academic files, goals and objectives, evaluations, policies, logs, and much more. If your TA asks you for documentation to support a site visit, make sure that you respond in a timely manner. Documentation is sent, in advance, to the RC Field Representative (commonly referred to as the "site visitor." Never call them inspectors). Then, on the day of the visit, the site visitor will have sessions with multiple stakeholders in order to ask questions and to clarify information that was in the prior documentation. It is common to have an hour session with the PD and TA, followed by an hour each with the faculty, residents, and DIO. The visitor is attempting to determine if the program is compliant with accreditation requirements and may ask the same questions of each group to see if their answers conflict or confirm the data previously given.

I recommend that you treat this as you would a court hearing. Answer the questions, but do not offer any further information than you must. Make sure you understand all the information we discussed earlier in this chapter. You should know your core competencies, how milestones are used, when and how you are evaluated, how this is documented, the types of supervision, what roles the faculty serve in the program, etc. Be cordial with the site visitor but realize that he/she is not here to discuss any issues that you currently have with the program. If you have any issues or complaints, make sure that you bring them to your PD, not to the visitor. The visitor is likely to report any complaints or discontent to the RC, which will not be helpful to the program's accreditation. The visitor creates a report from the visit notes and submits them to the RC. The RC reviews the report and decides on the program's accreditation status, based on this report and data provided in the program's annual reports to the ACGME. The same process happens for the Institutional RC when the sponsoring institution's accreditation is up for renewal.

CLER Visits

Clinical Learning Environment Review (CLER) visits are very different from RC site visits. The CLER occurs approximately every 18 months. There are normally three CLER visitors for this two-day event. It is an institution wide site visit with the GME department and hospital administrators actively involved together. The Chief Executive Officer,

Chief Nursing Officer, Quality Officer, Chief Medical Officer, and Graduate Medical Education Committee participate in multiple sessions of the CLER visitors. The remainder of the visit is spent with residents touring around the hospitals and clinics. They try to speak with as many residents as possible in the actual clinical learning environment, rather than in a conference room. This occurs over several different shifts, often observing patient handoff, morning reports, and rounds. The visitors will also stop nurses in the clinical areas to ask questions about residents' credentials to do procedures, communication between departments, and many other issues.

To prepare for a CLER visit, I recommend that all involved review the CLER Pathways to Excellence book published by the ACGME[20]. This book outlines the framework for patient safety and optimum education with six CLER Pathways listed as goals for improvements that each sponsoring institution should be striving to meet. The six focus areas are:

- Patient Safety
- Health Care Quality
- Care Transitions
- Supervision
- Well-being
- Professionalism

Scholarly Activity

Regardless of your specialty, you will be expected to participate in some form of scholarly activity throughout your residency. This can be in many forms. Some residents sit on hospital committees and work on

---

[20] ACGME, CLER Pathways to Excellence: Expectations for an optimal clinical learning environment to achieve safe and high quality patient care, Version 1.1 (2017). Found at: https://www.acgme.org/Portals/0/PDFs/CLER/CLER_Pathways_V1.1_Digital_Final.pdf

quality improvement projects. While others develop educational tools or processes for teaching students or underclassmen. Some specialties have higher standards and expect residents to be publishing peer review articles or book chapters. New residents often go through workshops to train them on how to develop a research question, design a study, process the documentation with Institutional Review Boards to get permission to move forward on projects, collect data, analyze data, write up the results, and submit for publication. This is an immense topic that cannot be addressed appropriately here. I wanted to bring this topic to your attention, to ensure that you are aware of the necessity to learn more about your institution's and program's expectations and procedures for moving forward. You may need to complete training in Human Subjects Research in order to do your required research. Check with your medical school or residency to see if they are a member of the Collaborative Institutional Training Initiative (CITI Program). Completing Human Subjects Research training in the CITI program is a good first step towards starting your scholarly activity. CITI also offers Medical Ethics courses and Research Design Courses.

Most sponsoring institutions will have, or are developing, a curriculum for research along with resources for residents to use in designing and implementing their projects. I recommend that you begin working with a resident while you are a medical student to start understanding the process. Then, when you begin your PGY1 year, team up with an upper classman that may already have a project in the works. You may be able to turn that project into a longitudinal project with minimum extra approval required. If you must begin a project on your own, use all the resources that are available to you and team up with someone if you can.

If you do not need to have a traditional research project, you may be able to do chart reviews that support quality indicators, a literature review summary for publication, or a process/quality improvement. If you are looking for a quality improvement project, the best question to ask yourself is - what process or situation bothers you and your peers the most? Is there redundancy in your process that you would like to eliminate? Do you wish you could educate your patients differently? Is your no-show rate at the clinic too high? These questions can get you started on the road to scholarly activity. Just remember to include all stakeholders in the project. That redundancy may be required by a legal or contractual requirement that you are not aware of. If you do not have this knowledge, you will not be successful in making improvements.

Tips from Other Physicians

In my many years of running new resident orientation, I have heard several physicians give suggestions to the new residents. Many of these physicians were talented well-revered leaders that moved on to roles as specialty board presidents and chief medical officers. There are a few tips that have stood out and that I have chosen to share with you. This may seem like a rag-tag list, but I believe that it symbolizes the importance of professionalism and communication. I hope that you will remember a few of these tips when you begin your residency.

- Communication is key to your success as a trainee, caregiver, team member, and professional.
  - Greet others when you pass them in the hall. Use the Hospitality 10/5 Rule – at 10 feet make eye contact and at 5 feet smile with your lips and your eyes, then verbally greet approaching guests and team members. You do not have to stop to talk. Just a friendly hello or have a great day. If someone looks lost, ask if you can help them. These simple things will make you friendlier and more approachable to peers and team members, while making patients and guests feel that someone cares. The power of a smile is immense.

- o Do not use your cell phone in public areas. If you are walking in the hall, do not look at your phone. Make phone calls in private areas or workspaces only. Use your hallway time to observe your surroundings, be intentional in greeting others, and reflect on your day.
- o Make sure that you do not let your phone pull your attention from a patient or colleague during a conversation.
- Be patient centered
  - o When you are rounding on a patient in a hospital room or the emergency room, always sit when you can. Come all the way into the room. Do not stand by the door with your hand on the doorknob. You want to provide them with a comfort level that you are there to really check on them and will take good care of them. You do not want them to feel you are in a rush, because they will feel that you are rushing their care and may miss something. This is important for your relationship with the patient and for patient satisfaction scores, which are highly important for financial reasons to your institution and soon to you as well.
  - o Let patients know that you care and will do your very best every day.
  - o Always ask if you can get them anything before you leave. They often will never want to bother the doctor with a small request but appreciate the offer. Sometimes, they really do need something that a staff member could address, if you mention it to them.
  - o Answer all of the patient's questions and make sure that the family has all of the answers that they need as well.
  - o Some physicians intentionally round when they know family members are less likely to be there. Don't be that

physician! The family needs to understand the current situation as well as the patient and often times the patient is incapable of sharing information correctly with the family. You would like to talk to the doctor, if it was your parent or child, wouldn't you? Give this courtesy to all families. This may even mean you stop back by when they are expected, if they were not here when you rounded. This is the right thing to do.

- Professionalism and Ethics
  - Hold yourself to a higher standard than others do.
  - Always do what is right even when no one is looking.
  - Never talk badly about others; they will hear about it.
- Take criticism and reflect on it in order to make improvements
  - Be open to feedback and allow yourself to be moldable – listen to everyone, especially the seasoned nurses – learn from them. They may save you from a horrible situation someday.
  - Keep your ego in check – you need to understand that you are a trainee and that you do not know everything. You will mess up and you will go through difficult situations. Make sure that you learn from those situations. Always look for improvements that you can make in your own life/wellbeing and in your professional career and the care you provide to your patients.

Chapter Nine:
Document Now – Do Not Wait

I could claim that proper documentation of your residency experience is just as important as learning medical knowledge. You can say that is ridiculous, but if you don't have the proper documentation at the end of your training, you will not be able to practice medicine. You will need to acquire a full license to practice medicine. You need to achieve board certification prior to your Board eligibility status expiration (as defined by your issuing Board). You will also go through a credentialing process with institutions where you wish to have privileges and with insurance companies that you wish to pay for your services. For all of this, you will need to provide documentation to prove your training and that you can practice independently. Even if you stay at the same institution that you trained, you will be required to provide this documentation. The type of privileges that you will be granted are dependent on the proof that you can provide to these institutions. You need proof that you had the necessary scope and volume of experiences.

If you don't have the proper documentation at the end of your training, you will not be able to practice medicine!

Primarily, the documentation that you will need is a comprehensive logbook of all your procedures, diagnoses, and/or clinic patient encounters. The required elements of your log will be determined by your specialty. For more information, check out the American Board of

Medical Specialties or the American Osteopathic Association for details on board certification requirements.

Board certification requirements are not always the same as ACGME requirements. The residency and fellowship programs will ensure that the curriculum of your program meets ACGME requirements. However, you may have requirements set by your specialty board that is not addressed in the ACGME requirements. You need to make sure that you understand the requirements of each and that you will meet both requirements by the end of your training program. The most common difference is with the number of procedures or clinical experiences.

A comprehensive logbook is needed AFTER your graduate residency.

It is very tempting to log your procedures and clinical experiences to meet the minimal number for graduation and then stop logging. After all, once you have met the minimum number, why continue to log, right? That is all that you needed to do in order to graduate or move to the next level of supervision. The reason to continue logging is often never shared with residents, until they are graduating and have insufficient logs. I have known many senior residents that have scrambled to review past medical records in order to reconstruct logs that they did not think they needed. The main reason for logs is not to graduate. Yes, programs use them to prove that you have the proper experience to move to the next level of training or supervision. The logs are used to show the ACGME that the program is providing the proper curriculum to the residents. The program uses the logs to show sufficient scope and volume of experience to support the number of residents that they have, or they wish to have, in the future. All of these are good reasons to keep logs, but the number one reason for you to keep a comprehensive log of all your experiences is that you will need it after you graduate. Yes, I said after you graduate.

Document Now

Your procedure logs and case logs are not just to get you through residency. After you graduate, you will need to prove your training was sufficient to practice medicine independently. You will use your logs to prove your current level of clinical competency to potential employers, to join the medical staff at hospitals, to sit for certification boards, to become credentialed with insurance companies, etc. If you learn one thing from this chapter, it should be that logs are extremely important for your future. It may seem mundane to log everything that you do each day, but it may be the difference between getting the job you want or not. This is because you need to be able to prove your experience in order to get clinical privileges. Every resident experience is not the same and it is your responsibility to provide evidence that you have the required training and experience for the role you are applying for after graduation.

Chapter Ten:
Becoming a Leader in My Program

As soon as you begin your residency, you should have teaching responsibilities with medical students. As you continue into your upper classman years, you will teach the lower classmen (often referred to as junior residents). You may be given additional administrative responsibilities in the program, such as developing the call schedules, setting up didactic speakers, and interviewing residency candidates.

You can be a formal or informal leader in your program. The formal leader is the chief resident. Each residency program will have at least one chief resident. General surgery identifies all fifth-year residents as chief residents. Internal medicine may have a graduate remain with the program for one year as a post graduate chief resident. Some programs will skip the most senior resident class to have a resident that is two years from graduation as the chief resident. The choice of chief is dependent upon the individuals interested in the position and their skill sets. Not all residents are capable of being a chief resident. The chief is normally appointed by the program director and this role may or may not be compensated with a chief resident stipend. This appointment is revocable if the program director deems it necessary. This can occur for many reasons, such as the chief becomes overwhelmed with the responsibilities, falls behind with his/her own academic status, or displays behavior unbecoming of the office.

Regardless of your position, you have the power to influence the culture of your program and improve educational programming for all your peers. You should participate in any leadership training or professional development opportunities that present themselves. Learn more about things that are important to your hospital and GME administration: quality improvement, patient satisfaction, professionalism, cost containment, and anything related to the business of medicine. Healthcare systems often have leadership classes for their leadership employees. Take advantage of these resources. You will not regret it later when you have more training in leadership than your peers. While you may not feel you will benefit from some of these classes now, you will find that it can be very beneficial for you in the future. I highly recommend conflict negotiation and communication classes. They will give you tools that you can use in residency and beyond. Most importantly, be open to mentorship and coaching from senior leadership, or an outside coach if you have the resources. This will help to expand your knowledge and develop your leadership skills.

Chief Resident Responsibilities

The chief resident role is different based on the needs of the residency and the interests of the program director. Chief Residents tend to perform administrative functions, such as but not limited to:

- Develop and edit rotation and call schedules
- Schedule and coordinate lectures
- Supervise residents and students
- Represent the program at required events and meetings
- Promote positive internal and external customer relations, by actively seeking quality improvement and customer feedback.
- Participate in staff meetings, committees, educational activities, special projects, and task forces.
- Lead residency team in effective planning and implementation of daily responsibilities and resident education.
- Serve as a liaison between the program, residents, GME office, and hospital officials

- Provide guidance and mentorship to junior residents
- Serve as a positive role model and advocate for peers and junior residents in all programs
- Evaluate the program and help with program strategic planning

As the chief resident, you <u>will not</u> be responsible for Remediation and providing discipline. If you have a resident in your program that you believe needs remediation or discipline, you must notify your program director. DO NOT PUT YOURSELF IN THIS POSITION! The program director will work in collaboration with the DIO on these issues. There are very specific human resource laws that govern this process and you need to rely on the experts to address these issues. Placing yourself into this process may put you in a very difficult situation and potentially legally place you at risk. Make sure you are always following institutional policies when you are dealing with resident misbehavior or lack of compliance. Do not provide your own version of justice such as adding call days or shifts to the schedule. This may have been acceptable in the past but can jeopardize your program if you do it without HR approval.

You can help your peers and your program by documenting any incidents that you feel may be of concern. If you are responsible for doing evaluations of underclassmen or student, please do not pass them from your rotations just to "get rid of them." Take your role as a preceptor seriously and hold those that you teach accountable to the standards that are set for the rotation. Otherwise, you are not doing anyone a favor. Failure to address issues and fail a student, as needed, causes a serious problem later and potentially jeopardizes patient safety.

It is these tough situations that tend to cause the most stress and anxiety for chief residents. Make sure that you check in routinely with your program director and share any issues that you are seeing. Ask for advice and be transparent with your director. If he or she is not sure how to proceed, one of you should follow up with the DIO for advice. This is a resource that you have at any time. Use it. You and your PD are not

117

expected to be HR experts, but you are expected to reach out to one when you are not sure about appropriate actions to be taken.

Program Evaluation Committee

As a leader in the program, you should get involved in the ACGME required Program Evaluation Committee (PEC). This committee requires at least two faculty members and one resident to annually review the program. This review includes a detailed analysis of resident performance (outcomes), faculty development, graduate performance, and program quality. A summary of the program's annual goals and relevant data points are provided to the GMEC for reporting in the Sponsoring Institution's Annual Institutional Report (AIR). Each program should have annual PEC meetings, but they are encouraged to meet more often to check on goal progress throughout the year. This committee is not looking at individual resident performance like the Clinical Competency Committee does, instead they are looking at the outcomes or metrics that the program has met for the year. Questions that the PEC should be discussing are:

- How is the program doing in PGY level and average over-all in-training scores? Are there curriculum changes necessary to address categories that are specifically lower than others? Has there been improvement in scores over the last year?
- Are faculty members involved in professional development as teachers? What development opportunities has the program provided and are faculty taking part in these opportunities? What new training will be necessary in the coming year?
- How are the graduates doing on their board examinations? If the program does not have 100% board pass rate, what can the program do to improve the rate? Is everyone provided the opportunity to attend a board review course? If not, should this

be a requirement? Does the program have the funding to provide this resource?

- Each institution will have its own Annual Program Evaluation format with specific metrics it will require the program to report. When reviewing the necessary metrics, where does the program fall short of expectation? How will the program address these issues?

It is advisable for the PEC to go through a S.W.O.T. analysis to evaluate the program's current status and develop new strategic goals for the next year. S.W.O.T. stands for Strengths, Weaknesses, Opportunities, and Threats. It is a good exercise for the program to annually survey the residents and faculty for their comments regarding the program's current strengths and weaknesses. While the ACGME already does this, the report provided to the program is often not as useful for this task as we would like. Next, ask the residents and faculty for what opportunities they would like the program to participate in. Are there resources that they would suggest we purchase or suggested changes to the curriculum? Last, the PEC needs to be aware of potential threats to the program. These tend to be outside influences that can harm the program or that the program will need to be aware of in their future planning process. This could be GME funding, insurance payment changes in the field that will drastically change the clinical experience, retiring faculty, and so on.

After all this data is collected and reviewed, the PEC needs to develop goals for the next year. It is advisable to develop two to three S.M.A.R.T. goals. Goals should be:

- Specific
- Measurable
- Attainable
- Relevant
- Time based

For more information on S.W.O.T analysis or S.M.A.R.T. goals, there are many reliable sources online. Each program will create their own process, but if yours does not have one yet, I recommend that you bring these tools to your PD for consideration.

Chapter Eleven:
Looking Beyond Graduation

Entering a Fellowship

If you wish to subspecialize, you will need to apply for a fellowship as you are entering your final year of residency. There are two types of fellowships. ACGME accredited and non-accredited fellowships. ACGME accreditation is often necessary for subspecialty board certification. If you train in a non-accredited fellowship, you may not be eligible for board certification. There are some individuals that choose to train in non-accredited programs, because they want the additional training regardless of board eligibility. In some instances, a subspecialty may be so new that there are no accredited programs because the ACGME has not recognized the subspecialty yet. Make sure to check on the accreditation of fellowships that you are interested in applying to; as you cannot assume that they are accredited.

Before applying for a fellowship, you should analyze the cost versus benefit of doing the additional training. Here are some questions to ask yourself:

- Is there any additional salary or billing upcharges that make this fellowship attractive?
- Can I get advanced board certification from this additional training?
- Will the additional board certification increase your overall salary to make up for the additional cost of living on a fellow's salary and delaying interest payments on your loans?

- Is there additional moving cost because the fellowship is in another location?
- Is my personal life at a point where additional training is reasonable?
- Do you have senioritis and just need to get out of training programs and start a practice?

Entering another training program can be a difficult decision. Do not make this decision without seriously considering all the positive and negative issues related to continuing your training.

Entering Practice

In the future, we will publish another book that will discuss in detail how to navigate the timeline from pending graduation to attending physician. It will provide more insight into what you need to do in order to be ready for that next step in your career. However, I must share some basic information here, so you can better understand the reasons you need to prepare now and learn more details about this later.

We have discussed the need to understand the board certification requirements as well as your graduation requirements. Once you obtain board certification, it is a lifetime commitment. In order to work within that specialty or subspecialty, you must maintain the Board certification in your practicing specialty and/or subspecialty throughout your career. This often means that you are either retesting in the subject matter or doing continuing medical education (CME) in your specialty/subspecialty. Specialty boards can choose to require both continuing education and retesting. It is important that you understand the expectation in the specialty that you wish to pursue. You will be responsible for meeting the requirements on your own.

While residency training is geared toward preparing you for board certification and the PD is required to communicate the Board's eligibility requirements to residents, there is nothing that requires the residency program to assist you in getting certified. However, the program is graded by the institution and the ACGME on how well the graduates do on the certification examination. This metric means that some programs will assist you with board preparation to ensure that you are successful. After you obtain your certification, you are solely responsible for ensuring that you complete the necessary continuing medical education credits to keep your board certification and ultimately your medical staff appointments.

When you are graduating, you will be faced with a decision to enter into independent practice or become employed by a hospital, health system or multi-physician group. Both the independent and employed practice models offer benefits and drawbacks. Most of you will either work for a healthcare facility or a physician group. Other options would include working in a facility that must have healthcare as part of their services, such as a jail, prison, or senior living center. In addition, you may choose to work for a university as a faculty member or a researcher. Except for a full-time researcher, all other positions would require clinical practice. In order to practice clinically, you will need board certification, a medical license, and privileges to see and bill for patient care.

Licenses

As a resident and fellow, you will begin with an educational license. You can move to a full license, after meeting the necessary years of training. Some residents choose to have a full license in order to moonlight (work medically outside of the training program during or after the PGY2 year). If you already have a full license in the state which you will practice, you will probably not need to do this step at graduation. However, most residents will not have a full license or will be moving to another state, where they are not currently licensed. If you are in this situation, it is important to apply early for a non-restricted or full medical license.   Each state will have its own requirements for a physician license. In general, you will need to apply for a medical license and a controlled substance license. The fees will be significant, and you will need to provide proof of training, USMLE or COMLEX-USA scores, and other items requested by the state issuing the license. I suggest that as soon as you know where you will practice, you immediately begin the licensing and credentialing process.

Credentialing and Privileging

In order to prepare for clinical practice as a physician, you need to understand the difference between credentialing and privileging. Credentialing is the process of collecting and verifying your qualifications as a physician. These credentials are obtained by a healthcare facility via primary source verification. The medical staff services or credentialing department will reach out to your residency to verify your training, your specialty board to verify your board eligibility, the state licensing board to verify your license, etc. They will collect documentation on licensure, education, training, experience, or other qualifications. In addition, to support your request for clinical privileges, you will be asked to provide documentation such as a case logbook , generally for the last 12-24 months. A list of common documents requested is found in Appendix B.

After your documentation is complete, the healthcare facility will review your file and determine the scope of practice or privileges that you may have in their facility. This is done in all types of organizations, such as hospitals, healthcare facilities, and physician groups. The governing body of the organization grants privileges based on the credentialing documentation and the services that they would like you to provide to their patients. You must work clinically within the scope of practice for which these privileges allow. Deviating outside of this scope of practice is a professional legal risk and can potentially place you at risk for dismissal from the facility. This credentialing and privileging process occurs every two to three years for each individual physician at each institution where the physician has membership and/or privileges, as required by federal regulation, accrediting body standards and Medical Staff Bylaws, Rules and Regulations and the associated policies and procedures.

Other Enrollments

In order to bill for patient care, you will need to be enrolled with third party payer insurance companies. In the event you are employed by a health system or hospital, the institution for which you work will walk you through this process. In addition, you will need to enroll in federal registrations such as Medicare Provider (PECOS), National Provider Identifier (NPI), and state specific provider registries. For example, in Michigan, there is a registry named CHAMPS (Community Health Automated Medicaid Processing System).

To avoid costly delays in your career, make sure you are applying for licenses, submitting credentialing packets, and enrolling in necessary physician databases several months before you graduate.

The important take away from this chapter is that you must prepare for entering practice well before you graduate. If you start these preparations well in advance, you may be able to walk right into a position as an attending physician. If you delay until you graduate, you may be waiting 60-120 days before you are fully licensed, credentialed, privileged, and enrolled with insurance payers with permission to see patients and bill for services.

We hope that you have enjoyed this career guide for residency. For more information on the transition from residency to attending physician and what you need to be successful on the medical staff, please refer to our next book in this series. You will find that the information we share will put you ahead of your peers. Our hope is that we can save you the frustrations that you peers will and have experienced.

Resources

Accreditation Council for Graduate Medical Education
   https://acgme.org/

American Board of Medical Specialties
   https://www.abms.org/member-boards/specialty-subspecialty-certificates/

American Medical Association – FREIDA Residency Database
   https://freida.ama-assn.org/Freida/#/

American Osteopathic Association
   https://certification.osteopathic.org/

Centers for Medicare and Medicaid Services (CMS) Medicare Learning Network, *Guidelines for Teaching Physicians, Interns, and Residents* (March 2018), https://www.cms.gov/Outreach-and-Education/Medicare-Learning-Network-MLN/MLNProducts/Downloads/Teaching-Physicians-Fact-Sheet-ICN006437.pdf

Collaborative Institutional Training Initiative (CITI Program)
   https://about.citiprogram.org/en/series/human-subjects-research-hsr/

Joint Commission: Ambulatory Care Program: The Who, What, When, and Where's of Credentialing and Privileging, https://www.jointcommission.org/assets/1/6/AHC_who_what_when_and_where_credentialing_booklet.pdf

Medical Student Resources
   https://www.accepted.com/medical/residency-personal-statements

National Resident Matching Program
   https://www.nrmp.org/

Acronym listing

ABMS – American Board of Medical Specialties

ACGME – Accreditation Council for Graduate Medical Education

ACLS – Advanced Cardiac Life Support certification

AMA – American Medical Association

AOA – American Osteopathic Association

ASO – American School of Osteopathy

BLS – Basic Life Support certification

CCC – Clinical Competency Committee

CMS – Centers for Medicare and Medicaid Services

CHAMPS – Community Health Automated Medicaid Processing System in the State of Michigan

CLER – Clinical Learning Environment Review

CME – continuing medical education

CMO – Chief Medical Officer

COMLEX-USA (or COMLEX) – Comprehensive Osteopathic Medical Licensing Examination of the United States

CV – Curriculum Vitae

DIO – Designated Institutional Officer

DO – Doctor of Osteopathy, graduate from USA Osteopathic medical school

ECFMG – Educational Commission for Foreign Medical Graduates

ERAS – Electronic Residency Application System

FMG – Foreign Medical Graduates

FMLA (or FML) – Family Medical Leave Act, often shortened to Family Medical Leave

FREIDA – Fellowship and Residency Electronic Interactive Database maintained by the American Medical Association

GME – Graduate Medical Education

GMEC – Graduate Medical Education Committee

H1-B – non-immigrant Visa for specialty occupations

HR – Human Resources Department

IMG – International Medical graduate

J-1 – Exchange Visitor Visa

MD – Medical Doctor, graduate from USA Allopathic medical school

MSPE – Medical School Performance Evaluation (Dean's Letter)

NPI – National Provider Identification

NRMP – National Resident Matching Program

ONM – Osteopathic Neuromusculoskeletal Medicine

OPP – Osteopathic Principles and Practice

OR – Osteopathic Recognition

PC – Program Coordinator

PD – Program Director

PEC – Program Evaluation Committee

PECOS – Medicare Provider registration database

PGY – Post-Graduate Year

PLA – Program Letter of Agreement

PRG – Program Year

QI – Quality Improvement

R# - Resident year

STD – Short Term Disability

TA – Training Administrator

TAGME – Training Administrator of Graduate Medical Education

TY – Transitional Year

USA or US – United States of America

USMLE – United States Medical Licensing Examinations

Appendix A:
ACGME Specialties and Subspecialties

Allergy and Immunology
Anesthesiology
    Addiction Medicine
    Adult Cardiothoracic
    Anesthesiology Critical Care Medicine
    Clinical Informatics
    Hospice and Palliative Medicine
    Obstetric Anesthesiology
    Pain Medicine
    Pediatric Anesthesiology
    Regional Anesthesiology and Acute Pain Medicine
Colon and Rectal Surgery
Dermatology
    Dermatopathology
    Micrographic Surgery and Dermatologic Oncology
Emergency Medicine
    Addiction Medicine
    Clinical Informatics
    Emergency Medical Services
    Medical Toxicology
    Pediatric Emergency Medicine
    Sports Medicine
    Undersea and Hyperbaric Medicine
Family Medicine
    Addiction Medicine
    Clinical Informatics
    Geriatric Medicine
    Hospice and Palliative Medicine
    Sports Medicine

Internal Medicine
    Addiction Medicine
    Adult Congenital Heart Disease
    Advanced Heart Failure and Transplant Cardiology
    Cardiovascular Disease
    Clinical Cardiac Electrophysiology
    Clinical Informatics
    Critical Care Medicine
    Endocrinology, Diabetes, and Metabolism
    Gastroenterology
    Geriatric Medicine
    Hematology
    Hematology and Medical Oncology
    Hospice and Palliative Medicine
    Infectious Disease
    Internal Medicine-Pediatrics
    Interventional Cardiology
    Medical Oncology
    Nephrology
    Pulmonary Critical Care
    Pulmonary Disease
    Rheumatology
    Sleep Medicine
    Transplant Hepatology

Medical Genetics and Genomics
    Clinical Biochemical Genetics
    Clinical Informatics
    Laboratory Genetics and Genomics
    Medical Biochemical Genetics
    Molecular Genetic Pathology

Neurological Surgery
    Endovascular Surgical Neuroradiology

Neurology
  Child Neurology
  Neurology
    Brain Injury Medicine
    Clinical Neurophysiology
    Endovascular Surgical Neuroradiology
    Epilepsy
    Neurodevelopmental Disabilities
    Neuromuscular Medicine
    Pain Medicine
    Sleep Medicine
    Vascular Neurology
Nuclear Medicine
Obstetrics and Gynecology
    Addiction Medicine
    Female Pelvic Medicine and Reconstructive Surgery
    Gynecologic Oncology
    Maternal-Fetal Medicine
    Reproductive Endocrinology and Infertility
Ophthalmology
    Ophthalmic Plastic and Reconstructive Surgery
Orthopedic Surgery
    Adult Reconstructive Orthopaedic Surgery
    Foot and Ankle Orthopaedic Surgery
    Hand Surgery
    Musculoskeletal Oncology
    Orthopaedic Sports Medicine
    Orthopaedic Surgery of the Spine
    Orthopaedic Trauma
    Pediatric Orthopaedic Surgery
Osteopathic Neuromusculoskeletal Medicine
Otolaryngology – Head and Neck Surgery
    Neurotology
    Pediatric Otolaryngology

Pathology
      Blood Banking/Transfusion Medicine
      Chemical Pathology
      Clinical Informatics
      Cytopathology
      Dermatopathology
      Forensic Pathology
      Hematopathology
      Medical Microbiology
      Molecular Genetic Pathology
      Neuropathology
      Pediatric Pathology
      Selective Pathology

Pediatrics
      Addiction Medicine
      Adolescent Medicine
      Child Abuse Pediatrics
      Clinical Informatics
      Developmental-Behavioral Pediatrics
      Hospice and Palliative Medicine
      Internal Medicine-Pediatrics
      Neonatal-Perinatal Medicine
      Pediatric Cardiology
      Pediatric Critical Care Medicine
      Pediatric Emergency Medicine
      Pediatric Endocrinology
      Pediatric Gastroenterology
      Pediatric Hematology Oncology
      Pediatric Infectious Diseases
      Pediatric Nephrology
      Pediatric Pulmonology
      Pediatric Rheumatology
      Pediatric Transplant Hepatology
      Sleep Medicine
      Sports Medicine

Physical Medicine and Rehabilitation
 Brain Injury Medicine
 Neuromuscular Medicine
 Pain Medicine
 Pediatric Rehabilitation Medicine
 Spinal Cord Injury Medicine
 Sports Medicine
Plastic Surgery
 Hand Surgery
 Craniofacial Surgery
Preventative Medicine
Psychiatry
 Addiction Medicine
 Addiction Psychiatry
 Brain Injury Medicine
 Child and Adolescent Psychiatry
 Consultation-Liaison Psychiatry
 Forensic Psychiatry
 Geriatric Psychiatry
 Hospice and Palliative Medicine
 Sleep Medicine
Radiation Oncology
 Hospice and Palliative Medicine
Radiology
 Diagnostic Radiology
 Interventional Radiology-Integrated
 Abdominal Radiology
 Clinical Informatics
 Endovascular Surgical Neuroradiology
 Interventional Radiology
 Musculoskeletal Radiology
 Neuroradiology
 Nuclear Radiology
 Pediatric Radiology
 Vascular and Interventional Radiology

Surgery
    Complex General Surgical Oncology
    Hand Surgery
    Pediatric Surgery
    Surgical Critical Care
    Vascular Surgery
Thoracic Surgery
    Congenital Cardiac Surgery
Transitional Year
Urology
    Female Pelvic Medicine and Reconstructive Surgery
    Pediatric Urology

Appendix B:
Credentialing Documents

A list of common documents generally requested for credentialing as a practicing physician:

- Legal/Official photo ID (copy of driver's license/passport)
- Immigration documents/green card if foreign medical graduate
- Proof of influenza, TB or other types of vaccinations
- Completion, in full, of credentialing application
  - Signed/date attestation statement as to accuracy of information submitted
  - Signed/dated consent and release form
- Completion, in full, of clinical privilege request form
- Copies of
  - USMLE/ECFMG certificates, if applicable
  - Medical School diploma
  - Internship/Residency certificate
  - Fellowship certificate
  - Board certification certificate or proof of Board eligibility from issuing Board
  - Current C.V.
  - State license(s) to practice
  - State Controlled Substance License
  - Federal Controlled Substance License (DEA)
  - Clinical case logs, which support clinical privileges requested
  - Current and previous professional liability insurance certificates of insurance
  - W9, showing Group Name/Business Name, Tax Identification Number (TIN) and associates billing address

Author Biographies

Sheri L. Clarke, PhD, C-TAGME

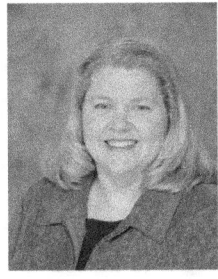

With a Bachelor's degree in Zoology from Michigan State University, Dr. Clarke spent over a decade in a clinical genetics laboratory, where she was a certified Clinical Laboratory Specialist in Cytogenetics. She has a Master of Public Administration/Health Care Administration emphasis from Western Michigan University and a Doctorate from the Eastern Michigan University College of Technology (Simulation and Education). Dr. Clarke's career in education began with classroom instruction and personal tutoring of medical students in genetics, before she transitioned to medical education administration at the program, hospital, and the institutional levels.

Dr. Sheri L. Clarke has 20 years of experience in Graduate Medical Education (GME) and medical school clerkship oversight. She has been a Designated Institutional Official (DIO) for a health care system, Associate Director/ Director of Medical Education for community teaching hospitals, and Chairperson of Graduate Medical Education Committees. She is the CEO and Senior Consultant for MedEd Associates, Inc.

Dr. Clarke serves as a Region Representative on the Board of Directors for the Association of Hospital Medical Educators (AHME). She has served on the Board of Directors for two educational consortia and was a long-time active member of a third consortium. Dr. Clarke was recruited to participate in the development of Training Administrator of Graduate Medical Education (TAGME) certification in 2003-2005, with the ACGME General Surgery Specialty. She led a task force in the creation of certification for central GME staff (2009-2012) and served on multiple TAGME committees, including the Board of Directors from 2002 to 2017. In addition, she is a past President and Treasurer of the Michigan Association for Medical Education.

Dr. Clarke is an Adjunct Faculty, for the Michigan State University College of Osteopathic Medicine's Department of Family and Community Medicine. She is actively working on her own research areas of interest (simulation, assessment, and GME administration) with over 25 oral and poster presentations at regional and national conferences in the past 15 years. She has won awards for her national presentations at both ACGME and AHME conferences. She serves as a judge for both oral and poster presentations at regional and state resident research forums.

Jodie M. Chant, MPA/HCA, BHSA, CPCS, RHIT

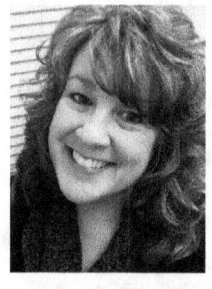

Jodie Chant possesses more than twenty-three years of health care experience, including nineteen years in administrative health care leadership in the acute care, managed care, and physician hospital settings. Jodie recently served as Health System Director of Medical Staff Services and Performance Improvement for a large health care system in Michigan, directing centralized credentialing operations for 5 hospitals and a health plan, medical staff accreditation and regulatory compliance, criteria-based privileging, medical staff peer review, institutional mortality review and all aspects of Focused and Ongoing Professional Practice Evaluations (FPPE/OPPE). Jodie also has experience in health information management, credentialing software development, provider enrollment and network management.

Given the numerous demands placed on our physicians from hospitals, insurers, and various state and federal regulations, Jodie has developed a passion to support and promote physician success, clinically and administratively. In 2016, Jodie started her own consulting and management services firm, Jodie Chant Consulting, LLC/Chant Medical Staff Resources, which provides clients nationwide with expert services and consulting in credentialing, delegated and centralized credentialing, privileging, accreditation and regulatory compliance, OPPE, FPPE, peer review, informatics and performance improvement, as well as physician organization executive management services, insurance payor contracting and member management.

Jodie graduated from the University of Michigan with a Master of Public/Health Care Administration, holds undergraduate degrees in Health Science Administration, Applied Science and is a former emergency medical technician (EMT). Jodie is a Registered Health Information Technologist (RHIT), a Certified Provider Credentialing Specialist (CPCS) and a TeamSTEPPS Master Trainer. Jodie previously served as President-Elect and President of the Michigan Association of Medical Staff Services (MAMSS) and served on numerous Committees with the National Association of Medical Staff Services (NAMSS). Jodie has authored numerous publications and given presentations on a variety of credentialing, privileging, peer review and physician/medical staff issues. Jodie is a current member of MAMSS, NAMSS, the American Health Information Management Association (AHIMA) and the Michigan Health Information Management Association (MHIMA) and serves as a member on the HCPro Credentialing Resource Center's Advisory Board, as well as a Member on the Tools and Forms Committee.

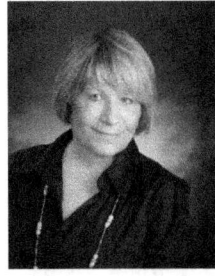

Rebecca Kraus, PCC

Rebecca Kraus has over 25 years of experience as an executive and physician coach, organizational development consultant and strategic planner. Rebecca possesses the unique ability to help her clients grow their leadership skills and emotional intelligence while strengthening their strategic business acumen. Her career work includes coaching, consulting and planning with over 300 administrative and clinical executives and their teams across multiple industries from healthcare to nonprofits and higher education.

She is the owner of Rebecca Kraus & Associates LLC, founded in 2006. Rebecca has designed and delivered customized administrative and physician leadership development programs for health care systems focused on building inspirational clinical leaders through the growth of emotional intelligence, communication and change management skills. As a certified physician coach, she has coached numerous physicians from surgeons to Internal Medicine and Family Practice. Her clients have spanned positions from clinical senior leadership (CMO's) to residents. Rebecca has designed and delivered numerous workshops for thousands of employees within healthcare on culture, communication, building teams, emotional intelligence, transparent leadership, conflict resolution, managing change and developing high reliability organizations. Rebecca has also designed and facilitated a hospital-wide patient satisfaction initiative involving over 1,800 clinical and administrative employees that resulted in drastically improved HCAP scores. She has also written and published many articles on leadership and behavior and is a popular presenter.

Rebecca is certified as a Professional Certified Coach (PCC) International Coach Federation (ICF) as well as a Mentor Coach. She is a Certified Physician Coach through the Physician Coaching Institute, and is certified as a professional Behavioral Analyst in DISC, PIAV, TriMetrix and 360 instruments. She has completed certification as a Social and Emotional Intelligence Coach through the Institute for Social and Emotional Intelligence.

Rebecca attended Michigan State University and is a BA dual-major graduate of Wayne State University, Summa Cum Laude and Phi Beta Kappa. She is a graduate of Corporate Coach U and the Planned Changed Internship Program created by Drs. Sylvia and Larry Lippett, professors from the University of Michigan. She has served as a Board member, Education and Development Chair and the 2015 State President of the Michigan Charter Chapter of The International Coach Foundation. She has been honored with the ICF Midwest Region Innovation Award by her peers for her work in developing a landmark continuing education training program for the state chapter that has been emulated by other state organizations.

Let's keep the conversation going...

We hope that Volume I of this series has helped you in being successful on your Road to Residency and Beyond. As you become a senior resident, make sure to use the next volume, *Physician Career Guidebook: Navigating the Chasm from Residency to Practicing Physician*.

Our Guidebooks provide you with a large amount of information across a wide range of topics. To dig deeper into any given topic, look for our corresponding *Physician Career Reference* e-books on Amazon. These Reference books will go into more detail on some of the topics we were only able to cover in a brief manner in the Guidebooks. If you would like further topics covered, share your questions with us.

We appreciate your feedback. Please share your story as to how this book was helpful to you in your career pathway, you can contact the author at SheriClarke@mededassoc.com or visit MedEdAssoc.com.

www.ingramcontent.com/pod-product-compliance
Lightning Source LLC
Chambersburg PA
CBHW070551220526
45467CB00003B/1165